EXPOSING
THE
SPIRITUAL ROOTS
OF
AUTOIMMUNE
DISEASES

EXPOSING

THE

SPIRITUAL ROOTS

OF

AUTOIMMUNE
DISEASES

POWERFUL ANSWERS FOR
HEALING AND DISEASE PREVENTION

DR. HENRY W. WRIGHT

WHITAKER
HOUSE

Publisher's Note: This book is not intended to provide medical or psychological advice or to take the place of medical advice and treatment from your personal physician. Those who are having suicidal thoughts or who have been emotionally, physically, or sexually abused should seek help from a mental health professional or qualified counselor. Neither the publisher nor the author nor the author's ministry takes any responsibility for any possible consequences from any action taken by any person reading or following the information in this book. If readers are taking prescription medications, they should consult with their physicians and not take themselves off prescribed medicines without the proper supervision of a physician. Always consult your physician or other qualified health-care professional before undertaking any change in your physical regimen, whether fasting, diet, medications, or exercise.

All Scripture quotations are taken from the King James Version of the Holy Bible.

Boldface type in Scripture quotations indicates the author's emphasis. The forms LORD and GOD (in small capital letters) in Bible quotations represent the Hebrew name for God *Yahweh* (Jehovah), while *Lord* and *God* normally represent the name *Adonai*, in accordance with the Bible version used.

Exposing the Spiritual Roots of Autoimmune Diseases
Powerful Answers for Healing and Disease Prevention

Be in Health®, LLC
4178 Crest Highway, Thomaston, GA 30286
www.beinhealth.com
info@beinhealth.com

ISBN: 978-1-64123-754-3
eBook ISBN: 978-1-64123-755-0
Printed in the United States of America
© 2021 by Be in Health®, LLC. All rights reserved.

Whitaker House
1030 Hunt Valley Circle New Kensington, PA 15068
www.whitakerhouse.com

Library of Congress Control Number: 2021948001

3 4 5 6 7 8 9 10 11 **W** 28 27 26 25 24 23

CONTENTS

DISCLAIMER

We do not seek to be in conflict with any medical or psychiatric practice, or any church or its religious doctrines, beliefs, or practices. We are not part of medicine or psychology; we are working to make them more effective, believing that many human problems are fundamentally spiritual, with associated physiological and psychological manifestations. This information is intended for your general knowledge only, to give insight into disease, its problems, and possible solutions. It is not a substitute for medical advice or treatment from specific medical conditions or disorders. We do not diagnose or treat disease.

You should seek prompt medical care for any specific health issues. Treatment modalities around your specific health issues are between you and your physician. We are not responsible for a person's disease or their healing. We are administering the Scriptures and what they say about this subject, along with what the medical and scientific communities have observed in line with this insight. There is no guarantee any person will be healed or any disease prevented. The fruit of this teaching will come forth out of the application of the principles and the relation-ship between each person and God. Be in Health® is patterned after 2 Corinthians 5:18–20, 1 Corinthians 12, Ephesians 4, and Mark 16:15–20.

FOREWORD

My husband, Dr. Henry W. Wright, was a brilliant man with a hunger for learning and an even stronger desire to serve God with all of his heart. He met the challenges of life with compassion, tough love, and his unique humor. It would be impossible to measure the impact he had on the lives of the people around him. His heart was to lead others to wholeness and peace in the love of God. He did his best to represent God's love in all that he did.

During his early years as a pastor, Henry's prayer was for answers to why physical healing from disease was not happening as often as it should in the church. That question, and God's answers, began his lifelong journey to exposing the spiritual roots of disease that were plaguing the body of Christ.

Henry spent decades researching biblical truths on what God said about healing, studying case histories of the people who came to the ministry for help, and learning about diseases and their effects on the human body from medical science. Together, we founded Be in Health and traveled throughout the United States and countries worldwide to teach biblical truths for overcoming diseases. The fantastic results were healing and restoration for tens of thousands of people across the globe. As the need for ministry increased, the For My Life Retreat was birthed. This impactful weeklong retreat on our church campus in Thomaston, Georgia, helps people understand the spiritual root causes of disease, apply the scriptural truths to their lives, and learn how to be set free!

Henry passed away in November 2019. Along with our family, church, and friends, I miss his presence every day. Shortly after Henry's passing, God spoke to my heart, "He's with Me, and he's good." Over five years ago, Henry and I, along with the Board of Elders, developed a plan to carry the biblical truths God had given him far into the future. Through Henry's relationship with the eldership and church body, we had a clear vision of how to move forward. Henry's vision was to establish generations of overcomers who would be restored—spirit, soul, and body—by God's Word and love.

Today, that is exactly what we are doing. The Be in Health team has expanded and continues to minister to thousands each month via our Thomaston, Georgia, campus, online seminars, mini-teachings, and conferences in cities across the country. The world is in great need of God's love and power to defeat the enemy and any diseases in their lives. I hope the biblical insights Henry deposited in this book help lead you in your journey of healing and restoration.

—*Donna Wright*

One

WHY AM I SICK?

Why am I sick?" "Why did this happen to me?" If you are fighting an autoimmune disease today, you are searching everywhere for answers to these painful questions. At Be in Health, I have spent decades researching the *root cause of disease*. This is vital because people want to know the answers: "Why am I sick?" and "How can I be well?" Doesn't it make sense that we get down to the *root cause* that triggers disease in the first place? From there we can uproot it! Why? Because it is God's desire for you to live in health and wholeness!

By God's grace, we have discovered answers to the root causes of disease that can put you on the road to healing and health. I want to state from the beginning that my research has revealed that approximately 80 percent of all chronic diseases have a *spiritual* root cause. Eighty percent is an astounding number! I believe that it is God's will to expose those spiritual roots and set you on the pathway to health. Because of what God has revealed in over thirty years of observing case studies, research into science, and studying His Word, thousands of people worldwide are free of their diseases and syndromes because they dealt with the root issues causing the manifestations. The healing answers that we will share now are from God's guidance and His Word, and all the glory for these healings belongs to Him!

GOD'S PROMISES FOR HEALTH

God has given us many promises for health and healing. He meant for us to live in wholeness. "[I am the God] *who forgiveth all thine iniquities; who healeth all thy diseases*" (Psalm 103:3). "*Who his own self* [Jesus] *bare our sins in his own body on the tree, that we, being dead to sins, should live unto righteousness: by whose stripes ye were healed*" (1 Peter 2:24). Jesus also declared that healing was the "*children's bread*." (See Matthew 15:26.)

If God has promised us that our diseases can be healed, then why are we sick? Why are so many people, including Christians, still suffering with chronic illnesses—autoimmune diseases such as multiple sclerosis, rheumatoid arthritis, lupus, Graves' disease, diabetes 1, as well as cancer, diabetes 2, high blood pressure and heart disease, chronic depression, and so many more? To find the answers, we need to take a journey together to expose the spiritual roots of disease and discover how you can live in wholeness—spirit, soul, and body. My prayer is that this journey will fill you with peace and produce the understanding and wisdom that will bring you freedom from your disease!

WHAT IS AUTOIMMUNE DISEASE?

Autoimmune disease takes a toll on the lives of millions of people in the United States every year. It is the third most common category of disease in the U.S. after cancer and cardiovascular disease, affecting more than 8 percent of the country's population or approximately 23.5 million people.[1] Over 80 different autoimmune diseases have been identified, and, for unexplained medical reasons, more than 78 percent of the people affected with these autoimmune diseases are women.[2] We know that autoimmune diseases can affect every biological system in the body, including the endocrine system, connective tissue, gastrointestinal tract, heart, skin, and kidneys.[3] I think that we can safely say that autoimmune disease is a "rising plague" in our culture today.

Autoimmune means "immunity against self." Science has discovered that your white corpuscles—which were designed by God to fight off disease—are identifying some healthy part of your body as an enemy invader and attacking it to destroy it. It is the body attacking the body. But doctors don't know why; they don't know what has gone wrong. In the medical community, the diagnosis of an autoimmune disease is a life sentence: there is no known cause and no known cure. The best that doctors can do is attempt to reduce or control your symptoms—not bring healing.

There is so much misunderstanding in the medical community and even in the church about the root cause of disease

1. National Institutes of Health: The Autoimmune Diseases Coordinating Committee: Report to Congress, *Progress in Autoimmune Diseases Research*, March 2005, https://www.niaid.nih.gov/sites/default/files/adccfinal.pdf.
2. DeLisa Fairweather, Sylvia Frisancho-Kiss, and Noel R. Rose, "Sex Differences in Autoimmune Disease from a Pathological Perspective," *The American Journal of Pathology*, September 2008: 173(3): 600–609, https://www.ncbi.nlm.nih.gov/pmc/articles/PMC2527069/.
3. DeLisa Fairweather and Noel R. Rose, "Women and Autoimmune Diseases," *Emerging Infectious Diseases*, November 2004, 10(11): 2005–2011, https://www.ncbi.nlm.nih.gov/pmc/articles/PMC3328995/.

in mankind. In my research, I have studied what God has said in His Word very closely, and I have also spent years studying medical science. It's important to study the human body God has created as well as what He has declared in His Word about our bodies and health. Although some people have accused me of being against medical science, I'm actually indebted to it because it has enabled me to see things that I could not see otherwise.

Unfortunately, the blind side of science is that scientists and medical professionals tend to believe only what they can perceive with their five physical senses. The Bible gives us a much greater insight to see beyond what we can observe in the natural. Answers to man's diseases and problems have been laid out in the Bible for over thirty-five hundred years. So why don't people read the Bible to discover those answers? That is what we are going to do in the following chapters. We will look at what God *and* science have to say about the root causes of and pathways to recovery from disease—especially autoimmune diseases. We will uncover the answers that you are searching for—to put you on the road to healing and health.

ARE AUTOIMMUNE DISEASES INCURABLE?

I want to put to rest those fears that you can never be cured of an autoimmune disease. With God, all things are possible! (See, for example, Matthew 19:26.) There is complete healing and restoration possible for all diseases—including autoimmune disease. By God's grace, at Be in Health, we have identified the spiritual roots of autoimmune disease and successfully helped people overcome those root causes with amazing results of healing and recovery. They have found the pathway to true, lasting healing that comes from God. According to Psalm 103, God heals all your diseases, redeems your life from the pit, crowns you with love, and makes you feel young all over again! That is the love of God! *"Who forgiveth all thine iniquities; who healeth all thy diseases; who redeemeth thy life from the pit; who crowneth thee with loving-kindness and tender mercies; who satisfieth thy mouth with good things; so that thy youth is renewed like the eagle's"* (Psalm 103:3–5).

Disease prevents you from a full life; healing gets you back to normal and maybe even better than you were before your diagnosis. That is *A More Excellent Way*! You will learn from God's Word how you can walk in healing and wholeness for the rest of your life!

CREATED IN HIS IMAGE

The Bible tells us in Genesis that God created man in His own image. *"And God said, Let us make man in our image, after our likeness…So God created man in his own image, in the image of God created he him; male and female created he them"* (Genesis 1:26–27). If we live as God designed us, we will be changed back into His image and thrive. We will function at our highest level. However, if we follow paths or ways of thinking about ourselves that are not in agreement with His plan, we lose our identity in God and may open a door to disease in our bodies. God is the author of what He has created: you. God is the sustainer of what He has created: you. So, if we dismiss God as part of the equation in our healing, what have we got? We have cut ourselves off from the source of our answer to the recovery and healing of disease.

God's desire as our heavenly Father is to form us back into our true identity as His children, in His image, and according to His nature. To understand who we are, we need to know who God is. First and foremost, He is our Father. Jesus was sent to the earth to restore our relationship with our heavenly Father. *"For if, when we were enemies, we were **reconciled to God by the death of his Son**, much more, being reconciled, we shall be saved by his life"* (Romans 5:10). First John tells us that *"God is love"* (1 John 4:8, 16). And we reflect God's nature within us when we manifest the fruit of the Holy Spirit in our lives. *"The fruit of the Spirit is love, joy, peace, longsuffering, gentleness, goodness, faith, meekness, temperance"* (Galatians 5:22–23)—all attributes of a loving God.

Psalm 139:14–15 tells us that God the Father thoughtfully and carefully designed and created each one of us: *"I will praise thee; for I am fearfully and wonderfully made: marvellous are thy works; and that my soul knoweth right well. My substance was not hid from thee, when I was made in secret, and curiously wrought in the lowest parts of the earth."* We are each designed with a specific personality, unique characteristics, and our own purpose and place that are prepared for us in His family if we will accept it. We were not created or called to be anyone other than ourselves. Each person needs to settle in their own heart that they are fearfully and wonderfully made in the image of God, not in anyone else's image. God does not make accidents.

KEEP TRACKING WITH US STEP-BY-STEP

In *Exposing the Spiritual Roots of Autoimmune Disease*, you will recognize the areas in life that can separate us from our identity as children of God. The Father wants to help us realign our hearts with His heart. We must learn to accept what He says about us as truth. In this journey of truth, we will answer many questions along the way. How can this loss of your identity in God the Father lead to disease? How did the spiritual roots of disease begin? What are the specific spiritual roots of autoimmune disease, and how have they invaded your life and brought debilitating pain?

In the early chapters, we will expose the unseen forces that trigger all disease from within and how you can overcome them. You will recognize the battleground that paves the way for disease, and how to apply the Word of God to receive victory! In the later chapters, we will expose the root causes of *specific* autoimmune diseases, highlighting the amazing case studies of people who have experienced healing from their diseases. That is what this journey is all about.

Since there is a great deal to learn about the spiritual roots of autoimmune disease, I will take you step-by-step to help you truly understand how you can walk in healing and wholeness for the rest of your life! Please don't try to get ahead of yourself. Read the truths in this book one step at a time. The Bible encourages us to learn by establishing a *firm foundation* and then building upon it *one precept* (guiding principle) or line at a time. *"For precept must be upon precept, precept upon precept; line upon line, line upon line; here a little, and there a little"* (Isaiah 28:9–10). Keep tracking with us closely throughout this journey—your freedom from disease may depend on it!

Two

WHAT IS THE SPIRITUAL ROOT OF DISEASE?

Did you know that you are a creative miracle of God? We have already recognized that human beings were created in God's image. God is a triune Being—Three in One—Father, Son, and Holy Spirit. In God's divine plan, He created us with three essential parts as well—*spirit, soul,* and *body.* The Bible states clearly, "And the very God of peace sanctify you **wholly**; and I pray God your whole **spirit** and **soul** and **body** be preserved blameless unto the coming of our Lord Jesus Christ" (1 Thessalonians 5:23).

"*May the God of peace sanctify you **wholly**.*" That word here is not H-O-L-Y. Even though the word *sanctified* does mean HOLY, the King James version of this verse says sanctified "*wholly*." W-H-O-L-L-Y. Completely, every part of us—*spirit, soul, and body*—sanctified and whole for His glory. You are a spirit, you have a soul, and you live in a body; you are a triune being. We need to understand this vital truth so that we can be healed and whole. How does this work?

First, we have a body. Our body is like our house—we live inside of it. Some of us have fancy roofs, some of us have thatched roofs, some have no roofs at all. We like to focus on the outward part—the body. You know there's nothing wrong with making our houses look nice. After all, we paint our homes, put shutters on them, plant flowers around them, and enjoy the beauty. We do the same thing with our bodies—we live in our bodies, and we often dress them up. The way our bodies feel impacts us powerfully. We focus on our bodies because that is what we experience with our five senses. So, the body is what we see, but it is only one part of our being.

Second, we have a soul. God created men and women with a soul. Our soul is comprised of our mind, will, and emotions. The way we view and experience the world with our minds and emotions is an integral part of who we are and has a significant effect on our bodies. We are greatly impacted at the soul level. Science has recognized this for a number of years with something called the mind-body connection. "The mind-body connection is the link between a person's thoughts, attitudes, and behaviors and their physical health. While scientists have long understood that our emotions can affect our bodies, we're just now beginning to understand how emotions influence health and longevity."[4] "Mounting evidence for the role of the mind in disease and healing is leading to a greater acceptance of mind-body medicine."[5] However, science doesn't recognize the third part of our being—our spirit—and that acceptance of the spirit-soul-body

4. Lakshmi Menezes, MD, "What Is the Mind-Body Connection?" Florida Medical Clinic blog, August 24, 2020, https://www.floridamedicalclinic.com/blog/what-is-the-mind-body-connection/.
5. Vicki Brower, "Mind-Body Research Moves Towards the Mainstream," EMBO reports, v. 7(4), April 2006, https://www.ncbi.nlm.nih.gov/pmc/articles/PMC1456909/.

relationship is key in the understanding of and fight against disease.

Third, we have a spirit. The most important part of our creation as humans is our *spirit*. This is the part of our human makeup that science doesn't recognize, and sometimes the church doesn't recognize it, either. The medical community focuses on our body, and they understand that we have a soul, but the spirit is ignored completely. Why is it important that we recognize the existence of this third part of our being? Because so many chronic diseases have their root cause or beginning in our spirits!

The biblical truth is that the *real* you is not your physical body, no matter how much you fix it up! Your body is just what you see with your five physical senses. There is so much more to you! God's Word reveals that the greatest impact on who we are is from within, at the *spirit* level. Our *whole* man—spirit, soul, and body—must be well to live in health. Now, I see three different perspectives on the root causes of disease: those of the medical community, of many in the church, and of the Word of God. We will look at these three different perspectives a little more closely.

WHAT DOES THE MEDICAL COMMUNITY SAY?

What does the medical community say about the root cause of disease? The truth is that doctors are at a loss for how and why many diseases begin. In medical textbooks, a large number of diseases are listed with the name of the disease, the body parts affected, the diagnosis, the prognosis, and the protocols. At the end of these journal entries, a specific medical phrase is inserted:

"etiology unknown." *Etiology* comes from the Greek and means "root cause" or "giving a reason for." The medical community knows they can see the disease, they can diagnose it, and they can track it, but they don't know or understand what triggers it.

All autoimmune diseases are catalogued as having an unknown etiology. That would include the more than 80 autoimmune diseases, including the most well-known ones: multiple sclerosis, rheumatoid arthritis, lupus, Graves' disease, Crohn's disease, and psoriasis. This is true for other non-autoimmune diseases, as well, such as chronic fatigue syndrome, fibromyalgia, and irritable bowel syndrome. With any disease that is considered incurable, the best the medical community can do is offer "disease management"—a combination of pills, therapies, or surgeries to keep the disease under control and hopefully extend the patient's life.

Please believe me—I am not against doctors or science! I have spent decades studying what medical science knows about the intricate human body that God has created. I am very thankful for what I have learned. But I do not want to just offer you "disease management"! By God's help, I want to expose the spiritual roots of disease and offer true health—spirit, soul, and body! That's because the God I serve—He represents your wholeness!

WHAT DOES THE CHURCH SAY?

Unfortunately, many Christians are often confused about healing and health. They know that the Bible gives us promises for healing, such as Psalm 103:2–3: *"Bless the LORD…who forgiveth all thine iniquities; who healeth all thy diseases."* But then they ask a very fair question, "Why aren't we seeing more people being healed?"

Christian leaders don't know the answer to this question, and so doctrines are created that contradict the Bible, such as the argument that "supernatural healing ended with the first apostles." Discouragement, doubt, and unbelief creep into the church. Without answers to the question of healing, some Christians simply resign themselves to illness. They even begin to ask, "Is God the one who brings disease? Is God just testing us or purifying us?" But that's not what the Word of God says! The Bible says that what God desires for us is *health and wholeness*.

The apostle John wrote, *"Beloved, I wish **above all things** that thou mayest prosper and be in health, even as thy soul prospereth"* (3 John 2). Now, I ask you, is there anything more "all" than *"all"*? John says he wishes for health above *all* things. Jesus Himself stated, *"I am come that they might have life, and that they might have it more abundantly"* (John 10:10). Abundant life includes freedom from disease. I want to be very clear here. I believe God's perfect will is not just to heal you. His perfect will is that you *don't get sick in the first place!* But if you are sick, then His healing is yours!

I ask people who are confused about God and health, "Why would God bring disease? Why would God destroy what He created?" God is not trying to destroy you! After He created Adam and Eve, He looked at them and proclaimed, "It is very good." (See Genesis 27–31.) He never said, "Look at those diseased beings that I just created!" No, God does not give us disease. In Hosea 4: 6, the Lord warns, *"My people are destroyed for lack of knowledge."* This verb in the Hebrew is written in the present tense, so it still applies to us today: *"My people are [being] destroyed for lack of knowledge."* God's people are suffering *in the present* because they don't have the knowledge that they need in order to be in health!

In the church, we need *wholeness* centers—places where we can be healed in our *spirit, soul, and body.* We shouldn't just farm our people out to a medical world that doesn't understand God and doesn't understand how He desires to heal us and make us whole. If we want this wholeness, we must recognize the truth of how God created us.

WHAT DOES GOD'S WORD SAY?

The Bible is clear! God wants to bring truth and freedom to us in our spirits, our souls, and our bodies. Again, *"I pray God your whole **spirit and soul and body** be preserved blameless unto the coming of our Lord Jesus Christ"* (1 Thessalonians 5:23).

In a world that questions whether truth even exists and often redefines truth as relative to personal whims, God's truth remains the same. It is His Word—the Bible. The Bible states that *all* of the Scriptures are God-inspired: *"All scripture is given by inspiration of God, and is profitable for doctrine, for reproof, for correction, for instruction in righteousness"* (2 Timothy 3:16). Since the Bible contains God's truth, then that is where we will find our answers for health and wholeness. That is where we will find the root cause of disease and how we may be restored to health.

Since the healing promises are given over and over again by God in His Word, why are so many sons and daughters of the Father suffering with as much disease as the rest of the world?

Have God's promises changed? Never. The promises of God give us the foundation and the faith to stand against disease. If you take the promises out of the Bible, what do you have? Nothing for your faith to believe with or stand on. Your faith comes directly from hearing God's infallible Word. *"So then faith cometh by hearing, and hearing by the word of God"* (Romans 10:17). You hear His Word, and faith rises within your spirit, and you embrace that faith. Faith is for today; faith is for right now. Healing and health are for right now.

Then what is the disconnect? If God's Word says that healing is the children's bread (see Matthew 15:22–29), that Jesus paid for the curse of sin on the cross (see Galatians 3:13), and that by His stripes, or wounds, we are healed (see Isaiah 53:5), then what has happened to us? Where have things gone wrong?

SEPARATION IS THE SPIRITUAL ROOT OF DISEASE

As I said earlier, after more than thirty years of research and experience with thousands of individuals, I am convinced that the root cause of about 80 percent of all chronic disease is spiritual. And that spiritual root is the direct result of separation in our lives on three very important levels:

1. Separation from God, His Word, His person, and His love

2. Separation from yourself by not accepting yourself and struggling with self-hatred, guilt, and shame

3. Separation from others by a breach in relationships

In the Bible, the First and Second Great Commandments are the foundation for this truth. When Jesus was asked which of the commandments was the greatest, He answered, *"Thou shalt love the Lord thy God with all thy heart, and with all thy soul, and with all thy mind. This is the first and great commandment. And the second is like unto it, Thou shalt love thy neighbour as thyself. On these two commandments hang all the law and the prophets"* (Matthew 22:37–40). With these two great commandments, God reveals the importance of love and acceptance without separation. First, love God Almighty with all of your being; second, love yourself because God created you in His love; third, love your neighbor with the same love as you love yourself because God created your neighbor, as well. When we don't obey these commandments to love, our disobedience brings on a critical separation that leads to the spiritual roots of disease and misery in our lives.

SEPARATION FROM OUR HEAVENLY FATHER

The first root of disease is separation from God. Mankind— that includes Christians—is diseased most of all because we are *separated from God, His Word, and His love.* We must realign ourselves with the Father, embracing the truth of His love for us. Jesus showed us the deep love of the Father by dying on the cross for our eternal redemption. *"For God so loved the world, that he gave his only begotten Son…"* (John 3:16). The Bible assures us of God's love: *"And we have known and believed **the love that God hath to us**. God is love; and he that dwelleth in love dwelleth in God and God in him"* (1 John 4:16). To be free and healed, you must believe God's Word that He truly *loves you.*

Unfortunately, "religion" has made God the Father seem unapproachable. It is easier to focus our love on Jesus as our Savior because He showed His love for us on the cross. People may feel more connected to Jesus. But Jesus came to this earth specifically to reconcile us to our Father—to take our sin upon Himself so that we would not be separated from the Father again. *"Now all these things are of God, who hath reconciled us to himself by Jesus Christ, and hath given to us the ministry of reconciliation"* (2 Corinthians 5:18).

It is the Father's heart for you to know how precious you are to Him. He refers to you as His beloved. *"Put on therefore, as the elect of God, holy and beloved..."* (Colossians 3:12). *"I will call them my people, which were not my people; and her beloved, which was not beloved"* (Romans 9:25). When Philip asked Jesus, *"Show us the Father"* (John 14:8), Jesus replied, *"He that hath seen me hath seen the Father"* (John 14:9). How Jesus taught, spoke, and acted was a reflection of the Father. That means it was the Father's love for us that Jesus healed the multitudes, rebuked evil spirits, fed the thousands, raised loved ones from the dead.

Sometimes we have a disconnect with God's love because our earthly father was not a good representation of the heavenly Father. Many of us stumble over the love of the Father because we never heard our earthly father say that he loved us. All around the world, people in our conferences have admitted that they never heard their father say those three simple words: "I love you." That was my personal experience as well. As a result, we have a problem understanding our identity as sons or daughters of our heavenly Father. We become fractured in our true identity.

This is a disease maker. You don't want to be separated from your heavenly Father for any reason.

One of the things I've done for years to help people deal with the damage done by an earthly father is to go through something I call The Father's Love Ministry. If you have never heard your earthly father say, "I love you," I'm asking you to just open your heart and receive these words for your life:

On behalf of the father that did not, could not, or would not—or maybe just didn't know how to—tell you that he loves you; on behalf of that father, I want to take responsibility for your life. On behalf of that father, will you forgive him for not telling you, "I love you"? I am so sorry for his silence and the junk and the hardness that may have injured you and left you feeling stranded on the inside when you needed him so much.

Now, on behalf of that father, I want to tell you these words for your life: "I love you. I am so proud of you. I am glad that you were born. And you are a good son; you are a good daughter."

Embrace these words with all your heart.

SEPARATION FROM OURSELVES AND OTHERS

"And the second [great commandment] is like unto it, Thou shalt love thy neighbour as thyself" (Matthew 22:39).

The second root of disease is separation from ourselves. I discovered that it is impossible to love yourself if you have not accepted the Father's love for you. I have seen thousands of people over the last three-plus decades battle intensely with self-hatred, self-loathing, self-bitterness, and guilt. Not accepting the Father's love and hating yourself instead is a deep-rooted lie from the enemy that carries with it many grievous diseases and disorders. If this is your struggle, you must learn to accept yourself in your relationship with God and love yourself as God sees you, not embracing the deception of self-hatred and guilt. God loves you! He declares it in His Word, as we have already seen. This will be a vital link on this journey to identify the spiritual root of disease.

The third root of disease is separation from others. This flings the door wide-open to spiritually rooted disease. Unforgiveness and bitterness can become a root deep inside you that defiles those around you and makes your body extremely susceptible to disease. The Bible warns us, "[Look] *diligently lest any man fail of the grace of God; lest **any root of bitterness** spring up to trouble you, and thereby many be defiled*" (Hebrews 12:15).

Bitterness is a deeply rooted sin because you consider yourself to be God in the situation, judging right from wrong and choosing not to forgive. It is an ugly sin that corrodes like acid, eating away at your soul. First it poisons the mind and then the body. Be kind to yourself. Make peace with your family members, church leaders, brothers and sisters in Christ, and anyone else who has injured or offended you. God commands it, and He knows that it will destroy your life if you live in unforgiveness and bitterness.

Now, if the root of 80 percent of chronic disease is spiritual, then 80 percent of all healing starts with *the restoration of our relationships with God, ourselves, and others!* How do I know this? Decades of the intense study of disease and thousands of case studies later, I have seen the successful result of applying the truths you are about to learn. We will unfold this restoration of our relationships to God, ourselves, and others in great detail as we continue on our journey to healing.

HEALED FROM DISEASE

Right now, I'd like to share the case history of a woman named Christine who came to us at Be in Health to find answers for her healing of Graves' disease.

Over sixteen years ago, I was diagnosed with Graves' disease, an autoimmune disease where your body attacks the tissue in your healthy thyroid as though it were an enemy. The result is an overactive thyroid producing too much of the hormone thyroxine. I struggled for fourteen years with Graves' disease, and I had five miscarriages because of it. During my "thyroid storms," when I was overcome with irregular heartbeats, tremors, anxiety, and confusion, I felt like I was losing my mind. My older children thought I was going crazy, too! I was so weak—no strength at all. At that point, it seemed like my life was coming to an end even though I was only in my early forties. I felt hopeless.

During the years I struggled with Graves' disease, I tried many avenues to be healed. When the doctors and endocrinologists couldn't find a cure, I turned to

alternative methods, including essential oils, naturopath doctors, and fifteen supplements that I would take
every day. The results were the same. I was incurable.

Thankfully, I had a friend who had been to a For My
Life retreat. One day, she told me, "I think you have a
spirit of fear." I didn't know what she was talking about,
but I was curious. I traveled from Colorado to the Be in
Health center in Georgia. I didn't expect to be cured;
I just thought they might be able to make me feel a
little better. But I was wrong. God had so much more
for me there. The whole restoration process of bringing
me back to the Father's love was intense. I struggled to
believe that I was God's beloved. I kept confessing it to
my family so that I could hear my own words. Once
I finally believed it for myself, that's when my healing
began to come forth speedily.

I left the For My Life retreat in March. In May of
that year, I had an appointment with my naturopath
doctor in Arizona who had been running all of my blood
tests. The doctor was astonished at my test results.
She walked back into the examination room and said,
"Christine, I don't know what you've done, but your thyroid is totally normal! Your TSH (thyroid-stimulating
hormone), T3, and T4 hormone levels are all normal!"
The doctor ordered a new ultrasound, and my goiter
had disappeared completely! I had spent thousands of
dollars traveling to clinics, experimenting with natural
remedies, and taking those fifteen daily supplements

over the years. My healing came with no medications, no supplements! My greatest blessing? I had a baby at the age of forty-six! He's the perfect addition to our family!

I have seen true restoration in my life. God didn't just hand me back the years I lost; He greatly restored those years to me. I feel full of life. I feel younger than I have for years and have so much more energy than I ever did—and an abiding peace and joy. The main thing, truly the overriding message, has been the restoration with my heavenly Father. I really know that I am His beloved.

—Christine

Three

WHERE DISEASE BEGAN

In all three of the spiritual separations that we just read about, we are tempted by an unseen enemy to reject our love for God, ourselves, and others. This unseen enemy who finds a place to sneak in to destroy us is Satan, whom Jesus called *"the thief… [who comes] to kill, to steal, and to destroy"* (John 10:10). The apostle Paul warns us not to be *"ignorant of [Satan's] devices"* (2 Corinthians 2:11). The word *"devices"* refers to the devil's methods, mythologies, and practices—the way he has been scheming to destroy God's people since the garden of Eden. When you embrace the enemy's lies, you end up suffering at his hands. You need to know how the enemy is doing it. You need to understand his devices so that you can cut him off at the pass in your life! We need to look at how this happens and how disease began in the first place.

Do you know how many diseases there are? Over three thousand diseases and disorders have been identified to date! Where did they come from? They didn't come from God. When He created man, He created something that was very good, but then something came along to interfere—something that wasn't good. This is the enemy lurking around, whose sole ambition is to interfere with God's plan and destroy the people God has created. His name is Satan, and the goal of his dark kingdom is to steal, kill, and destroy God's people on earth.

HOW DISEASE ENTERED THE WORLD

Let's start at the beginning—with Adam and Eve.

According to Genesis, chapter two, Adam walked in the cool of the evening with his Creator before Eve came on the scene. Just before Eve was created, Adam was given the first law from God. *"And the LORD God commanded the man, saying, Of every tree of the garden thou mayest freely eat: but of the tree of the knowledge of good and evil, thou shalt not eat of it: for in the day that thou eatest thereof thou shalt surely die"* (Genesis 2:16–17).

In the garden of Eden, Satan, the great deceiver, came to Eve and changed the Word of God. *"Now the serpent was more subtil* [deceitful] *than any beast of the field which the LORD God had made. And he said unto the woman, Yea, hath God said, Ye shall not eat of every tree of the garden?"* (Genesis 3:1). In other words, "Is this what God really said?" When Eve replied that God said they would die if they ate the fruit of one specific tree, Satan lied to contradict God's Word. *"And the serpent said unto the woman, Ye shall not surely die: for God doth know that in the day ye eat thereof, then your eyes shall be opened, and ye shall be as gods, knowing good and evil"* (Genesis 3:4–5). In other words, he whispered the great deception we still hear today: "God lied to you...there's really a better plan."

You know what happened next. Eve broke off the fruit, ate it, and then handed it to her husband who was standing right beside her. She repeated the enemy's lie— "Adam, we won't die; our eyes will be open to good and evil. It's going to make us wise!"—and he ate. Immediately, their spiritual eyes were opened; but at that moment, wisdom didn't flood them—evil did. They saw their nakedness before a holy God, and they hid from Him in fear. Adam, son of God, was suddenly afraid of the One whom he had walked with in perfect fellowship.

As evening approached, it was time for the Lord to meet with them. Genesis chapter three tells us that the Lord came looking, calling out something like this: "Where are you, Adam?" Adam finally had enough nerve to answer, "Here we are, Lord! Out here in the bushes." "Why are you hiding from Me, Adam?" "Because, Lord, we are naked." Now, read the words of the Lord in Genesis 3:11: *"And he* [God] *said, Who told thee that thou wast naked?"* God knew why they were hiding. He knew it was Satan who had seduced Adam and Eve and was now overwhelming them with thoughts of fear, guilt, and shame. But He wanted to know if Adam knew who had come to destroy him and his perfect communion with God.

This was the beginning of Adam and Eve's journey into a life of temptation and sin. When Adam and Eve rebelled and disobeyed the first law of God, sin and death—both spiritual and physical—entered the world. Death and disease came to this planet because of their disobedience. As a result, sin, disease, and death have passed from generation to generation, and we are still battling them to this day. This is the origin of disease.

Thank God that He had a plan to save us from what Satan meant for our total destruction. He had a plan through His Son Jesus to redeem a people who would love Him. God gave us a plan for our eternal salvation through the death and resurrection of Jesus Christ. He also gave us a plan to defeat Satan's schemes in our lives on earth. So why aren't Christians always following the plan?

THERE ARE TWO KINGDOMS

This account of Adam and Eve reveals a vital biblical truth: disease is no happenstance; it is a planned event by our spiritual enemy, Satan, and his dark kingdom. Many Christians have forgotten that we have a hidden enemy who is after our destruction. Remember the Scripture verse that says, *"My people are destroyed for lack of knowledge"* (Hosea 4:6)? God wasn't speaking just to the Old Testament saints here. I see this same lack of knowledge in the modern church today. People are ignorant of spiritual warfare.

The spirit world is a place where intelligent beings exist that do not have bodies in a physical sense. There are two kingdoms in this invisible world. There is the kingdom of God, which the Father rules from heaven. Heaven is not far away; it's just on the other side of what we can see, in a different dimension. Then there's the kingdom of darkness, which is inhabited by fallen spiritual beings and ruled by the ex-Archangel, Satan. That kingdom may not seem real in our "modern age," but it is clearly defined in the Bible for our benefit.

Jesus spoke with a great awareness of this evil kingdom when He said, *"And if Satan cast out Satan, he is divided against himself; how shall then his kingdom stand?"* (Matthew 12:26). Jesus accused the Pharisees of siding with evil: *"Ye are of your father the devil, and the lusts of your father ye will do. He was a murderer from the beginning, and abode not in the truth, because there is no truth in him. When he speaketh a lie, he speaketh of his own: for he is a liar, and the father of it"* (John 8:44).

The apostle Paul also warned us that our battle in life is not against flesh and blood that we can see. *"For we wrestle not against flesh and blood, but against principalities, against powers, against the rulers of the darkness of this world, against spiritual wickedness in high places"* (Ephesians 6:12). Your war is not with others. Your war is not even with yourself. Your war is with an evil kingdom filled with principalities, powers, spiritual wickedness in high places, and the rulers of the darkness of this world that you cannot see with your physical eyes.

Just like Adam and Eve, your war is with a hidden enemy who wants to form you into his image, but that image is the image of disease and death. Adam and Eve embraced that image. Jesus Christ's image is the image of wholeness and life. You must learn to embrace Jesus and His image! It is vital to our lives and our health that we understand the biblical truth that two kingdoms exist in the spiritual world: one of darkness and one of light. Jesus sent Paul to the people *"to open their eyes, and to turn them from darkness to light, and from the power of Satan unto God"* (Acts 26:18). There is great warfare between these two kingdoms. When we don't understand what is going on in the spirit world, we become victims of our own ignorance.

YOU ARE NOT YOUR DISEASE!

Don't embrace the spirit of death. God has created you with a purpose and a plan. God has created you to live. It is the enemy who wants to overthrow the plan that God has created for you. *You are not your disease.* Remind yourself: "I may *have* a disease, but I *am not* a disease!" Don't call it "my disease." There is sin that has been tormenting you, but you are not the sin. You are a child of God! Accept the Father's great love for you; He has called you to be His own! *"Yea, I have loved thee with an everlasting love: therefore with lovingkindness have I drawn thee"* (Jeremiah 31:3). You are not the problem; the devil is. Stop listening to him!

My desire is to open your eyes to God's truth concerning the spiritual root of all disease and the freedom from disease that can be yours. I want you to join me in this walk of freedom. I want you to embrace life! I want you to defeat everything that God hates. I don't want to offer you a counterfeit of humanism. I want to offer you the truth from God's Word. *"Ye shall know the truth, and the truth shall make you free"* (John 8:32). I want you to live in freedom from the bondage and the curse of disease. Satan may have evil devices, but God shows us how we can defeat him and be in health.

HOW DO WE CHOOSE LIFE?

"I have set before you life and death, blessing and cursing: there-fore choose life" (Deuteronomy 30:19). Moses presented this deci-sion to God's people thousands of years ago, and we must make this same decision today—the choice between life and death,

blessings and curses. During his final address to the Israelites, Moses shared this powerful message from God. *"I call heaven and earth to record this day against you, that I have set before you **life and death, blessing and cursing**: therefore choose life, that both thou and thy seed may live"* (Deuteronomy 30:19).

Life and blessings come from obedience to God. *"And it shall come to pass, **if thou shalt hearken diligently** unto the voice of the LORD thy God, to observe and to do all his commandments which I command thee this day, that the LORD thy God will set thee on high above all nations of the earth. And **all these blessings** shall come on thee, and overtake thee, if thou shalt hearken unto the voice of the LORD thy God"* (Deuteronomy 28:1). Look what God was promising! If they chose God's voice—*if they chose life*—they would be *"high above all nations of the earth,"* and they would be *"overtaken"* by more blessings than they could count. These blessings would overtake them *if* they listened to and obeyed the Lord. What a promise!

However, that was not the end of Moses's message. He followed it with a warning that the Israelites should never forget. *"But it shall come to pass, **if thou wilt not hearken** unto the voice of the LORD thy God, to observe to do all his commandments and his statutes which I command thee this day; that **all these curses** shall come upon thee and overtake thee"* (Deuteronomy 28:15). For the next forty-three verses, Moses described the curses—the disastrous events and diseases—that would overtake God's chosen people if they chose not to listen to Him and not to follow His commandments. By their disobedience, they would open themselves to the enemy's lies, which would lead to curses...and many of those curses are diseases.

Please understand me—I am not into legalism. I am into something called heart change. I'm into understanding the Word of God because it is truth—truth that brings us freedom from disease. Some people say that the Old Testament is not for Christians today. However, in the Old Testament, God says that He will bless *"them that love me and keep my commandments"* (Deuteronomy 5:10). In the New Testament, Jesus said to His disciples, *"If ye love me, keep my commandments"* (John 14:15.) The apostle John wrote, *"For this is the love of God, that we keep his commandments: and his commandments are not grievous"* (1 John 5:3). Throughout the Bible, God asks us to obey His commandments because it is His will, and also because those commandments have been created for our good, our protection, and our health.

WHAT EXACTLY IS A CURSE?

Disobeying God can bring a curse of disease. What exactly is a curse? People are afraid of the word, and it isn't something we talk about much in the church today. I decided to do a little word study of the Hebrew word for *curse* based on Deuteronomy 28. The first word I found for the meaning of curse was *vilification*. Vilification starts with the same letters as the word *villain*. The minute I saw the word *villain*, I thought of Jesus's words about Satan. Jesus said, *"The thief cometh not, but for to steal, and to kill, and to destroy: I am come that they might have life, and that they might have it more abundantly"* (John 10:10). That thief—Satan— is the enemy, the villain in our lives. My study also revealed that a curse is *an abatement* of the blessing. The word *abatement* means "lessening" or "reduction." So, the villain, who is Satan, comes to abate or reduce the strength of our blessings from God. The curse is the work of this villain.

In Moses's address to the Israelites in Deuteronomy, chapter twenty-eight, we can find every class of disease known to man. God called these diseases the result of a curse—an abatement of His blessing. In my ministry, I began to encounter far too many New Testament believers who were plagued with the exact same diseases as those listed in Deuteronomy. They had autoimmune disease, they had heart disease, they had digestive disorders, they had cancer, they had depression. I began to wonder, "Why are these biological and psychological disorders called a curse in the Old Testament, but the same things that are found in New Testament covenant saints aren't called a curse?"

CAN CURSES AFFECT CHRISTIANS TODAY?

I am very serious about this. Our world, and even the church, is filled with every work of the devil found in Deuteronomy 28 which is called the curse. Disease, syndromes, depression, anxiety disorders, family discord, job loss—it's all there. Our lives are under attack, not just our bodies. That brings up an important question: Can curses affect Christians today? The Bible tells us that a curse without cause—without a reason for being there—cannot affect us. *"As the bird by wandering, as a swallow by flying, so a curse without cause shall not alight"* (Proverbs 20:2).

Didn't Christ end the curse from Adam and Eve by His death on the cross? *"Christ hath redeemed us from the curse of the law, being made a curse for us"* (Galatians 3:13). Yes, He did, and He made it possible for us to live in righteousness and wholeness by His death and resurrection. Then how can Christians, who are covered by the blood of the Lamb, be under the burden of a curse? It is because the effects of a curse are *a result of disobedience to God's Word*, and Christians can be just as disobedient to God's Word as the Old Testament believers were. Curses can alight because we give them the permission to do it!

Now, I am not talking about Christians being possessed by an evil spirit. I am not talking about losing your salvation. I am talking about servitude to the enemy. It means that you are serving the law of sin presented to you by Satan rather than serving the law of God. A curse that has no cause cannot affect a Christian's salvation. But it can wreak havoc in our lives if we give the villain who is behind that curse permission. Satan doesn't have all power. He can only touch you with your permission when you embrace the law of sin. How can we give the devil this permission? *By disobeying God and His Word and obeying the law of sin instead*. But God has provided the pathway to our freedom from the law of sin.

God's thinking is superior, and Satan's thinking is inferior. *"Ye are of God little children and have overcome them; because greater is he that is in you, than he that is in the world"* (1 John 4:4). Greater is God who is in you than the enemy who is in the world. You choose whom you will serve. God will not leave you or forsake you as you take this journey to freedom! Keep on tracking with me on this road to your health and wholeness. *"Be strong and be of good courage; fear not, nor be afraid of them: for the LORD thy God, he it is that doth go with thee; he will not fail thee, nor forsake thee!"* (Deuteronomy 31:6). Don't be afraid of this battle. God is our victory!

Four

WINNING THE WAR WITHIN

Did you know that as Christians we can still have a war raging within? Paul, an apostle of Jesus Christ, confessed that there was a war within him—two laws battling for his soul—the law of God and the law of sin. Paul declared:

> For the good that I would I do not: but the evil which I would not, that I do. Now if I do that I would not, it is no more I that do it, but sin that dwelleth in me. I find then a law, that, when I would do good, evil is present with me. For I delight **in the law of God** after the inward man: but I **see another law in my members**, warring against the law of my mind, and bringing me into **captivity to the law of sin** which is in my members. O wretched man that I am! who shall deliver me from the body of this death? **I thank God through Jesus Christ our Lord**.   (Romans 7:19–25)

PAUL'S WAR WITHIN

The battle between the law of sin and the law of God that happened in Paul two thousand years ago is still happening in us today. You may ask, "I thought we weren't under the law anymore?" When Paul talks about the law of God here, he isn't speaking about rules; he is referring to God's nature. It is a reflection of God's righteousness. God is good; God is love; God is justice; God is mercy; God is forgiveness; God is faithfulness. These things and more are His nature and His righteousness—the law that God promised to write on our hearts. *"I will put my laws into their mind, and write them in their hearts: and I will be to them a God, and they shall be to me a people"* (Hebrews 8:10).

On the other side of the war is the law of sin, which is the nature of Satan: rebellion, lawlessness, hatred, murder, evil, and falsehoods. The law of sin will always attempt to compete with the law of God through temptation. In this battle, Paul is saying, "The things that I wish I wouldn't do, that's what I do; and the good that I want to do, I don't do it." Well, that sounds just like us, doesn't it? How often do you find that there's an interference in your journey from all kinds of things, circumstances, thoughts, temptations, and who knows what else? The apostle Paul identifies with you. As an apostle, he had his own journey of overcoming. He shared it with us when he confessed that sometimes he did the very things he didn't want to do.

When he says, *"If then I do those things **that I would not do**,"* Paul is basically saying, "If I practice unforgiveness, it overtakes me. I hate it. I know I should always forgive, but for some reason I find myself holding grudges and records of wrongs and practicing unforgiveness. I hate unforgiveness, but I can't stop myself from *practicing* unforgiveness." It is the same as saying that the law of God—the law of forgiveness—is evil, and the law of unforgiveness is good. So, these two laws are battling inside you. The law and nature of God brings you health. The law of sin and nature of Satan brings you disease. The question for you to consider is this: Which law are you being influenced by today?

THE SNARE OF THE ENEMY

Over thirty years ago, when I asked the Lord why I didn't see more healing in my ministry as a pastor, God led me to 2 Timothy 2:24–26:

> *And the servant of the Lord must not strive, must be gentle unto all men, patient, apt to teach in meekness instructing those that oppose themselves; if God peradventure will give them repentance to the acknowledging of the truth; and that they may recover themselves **out of the snare of the devil, who are taken captive by him at his will**.*

Whoa, what? *"Recover themselves out of the snare of the devil"* and *"who are taken captive by him at his will!"* "Lord," I prayed, "this letter is written to Christians; how can this be happening?" My eyes were opened when I realized what Paul was saying. His words reveal that there can be something in a Christian's life that gives the devil a legal right to take them captive, to steal their blessings, and to put disease on them. I want to remind you that not all disease comes to people in this way. Not every disease has a spiritual root of sin, but I have found without question that a large portion of the chronic diseases that I have confronted have a spiritual root.

Jesus linked the law of sin and healing more than once in the New Testament. When He met the paralyzed man lying beside the pool of Bethsaida, Jesus healed the man by telling him to take up his bed and walk. Hours later, they met again in the temple. This time, Jesus told that same man that now that he was healed, he should go and sin no more, or something much worse would happen to him. *"Afterward Jesus findeth him in the temple, and said unto him, Behold, thou art made whole: sin no more, lest a worse thing come unto thee"* (John 5:14). Disease had come to this man through the law of sin; Jesus encouraged him to sin no more.

Other times, Jesus used both the phrases "you are healed" and "your sins are forgiven" when He healed someone. Matthew 9:1–5 and in Mark 2:5–10 record the same healing. *"And, behold, they brought to him a man sick of the palsy, lying on a bed: and Jesus seeing their faith said unto the sick of the palsy; Son, be of good cheer; thy sins be forgiven thee"* (Matthew 9:2). And the man was healed; he got up and walked. As we can see from the Scriptures, there can definitely be a connection between sickness and the law of sin in our lives.

REPENTANCE IS NOT A BAD WORD

> *That God peradventure will give them **repentance** to the acknowledging of the truth that they may **recover themselves from the snare of the devil**, who are taken captive by him at his will.* (2 Timothy 2:25–26)

Paul shared this Word with us because when we know the truth of God's law, of God's true nature, it brings us to *repentance.* Now, repentance is not a bad word. It doesn't mean that you are not a Christian or that you are an evil person. Paul was speaking to New Testament believers when he talked about this repentance. Can you imagine going to the Father, the Lord of creation, and saying, "Dad, I'm sorry. I come to You in Jesus's name, Father. I yielded to Satan's law of sin. I've been following it, but I hate it. I don't want to do it anymore. As it says in Your Word, it's not good for me. I come to You to take responsibility for my sin, and I repent to You for allowing it to control my life. Will You please forgive me?"

Is that hard? Oftentimes, we need to deal with sin and spiritual issues that are affecting our hearts before our healing can occur. That is a prescription directly from heaven, and it may save you from incurable diseases! Folks, you can do a lot to prevent disease in your life. Read these truths carefully and embrace them. We're so busy chasing symptoms and disease profiles that we don't take into account why we got sick in the first place.

We experience *repentance* from our sins when we first turn to God to acknowledge Jesus Christ's death and resurrection on our behalf. That is our *salvation.* Now, it would be great if, once we became Christians, we never sinned again. But that isn't what happens. Thank God that even when we do sin, and then confess it to God, He is always gracious to forgive us. *"If we say that we have no sin, we deceive ourselves, and the truth is not in us. If we confess our sins, he is faithful and just to forgive us our sins, and to cleanse us from all unrighteousness"* (1 John 1:8–9).

Sanctification also plays an important role in our becoming free from disease. As Christians, we need further repentance for things in our lives that aren't of God. That is our *sanctification.* Sanctification is a lifelong process for the Christian where, through the glories and trials of life, and through our obedience to Him, we learn to walk in the newness of life. *"That like as Christ was raised up from the dead by the glory of the Father, even so we also should walk in newness of life"* (Romans 6:4). Sanctification is God's plan for us. Our part is to embrace His truth, repent of any part of the law of sin, and allow Him to transform us into His image.

IT'S CONVICTION, NOT CONDEMNATION!

Please don't react to God's truth about sin in your life by condemning yourself. The Holy Spirit reveals our sins to us in order to bring repentance and freedom, not to condemn us! His conviction helps us recognize our sin so that we can repent and walk in the freedom of Jesus Christ. *"There is therefore now no condemnation to them which are in Christ Jesus, who walk not after the flesh, but after the Spirit"* (Romans 8:1). This is all the process of our sanctification, of our being changed as we grow in Him.

Our greatest encouragement is that the Holy Spirit is there to help us through the whole sanctification process. The Bible tells us, *"But we all, with open face beholding as in a glass the glory of the Lord, are changed into the same image from glory to glory, even as by the Spirit of the Lord"* (2 Corinthians 3:18). The words *"are changed into the same image"* are in the present progressive tense. That means that being changed into Christ's image is an ongoing process; we become more like Christ as we walk out our sanctification throughout our lives.

I do want you to understand that God is not going to live your life for you. That is why God gives you the responsibility of believing the truth of the Word when it comes to the battle with the law of sin. You must take ownership in this victory; you must activate; you must decide to wake up, be an overcomer, and face the things from the enemy in your life and defeat them in Jesus's name. Embrace the process of sanctification from God so that you can walk in the freedom of Jesus Christ!

UNFORGIVENESS AND DISEASE

Nearly twenty years ago, *Newsweek* magazine featured an article that startled the scientific community.[6] Research was uncovered that forgiveness and unforgiveness affect human health. When medical science discovered this truth, they declared that unforgiveness was a disease. They named it a disease because they recognized its effect on the human body. However, that's not what the Bible calls it. The Bible calls unforgiveness sin.

Our biggest problem in overcoming disease is that people want to be healed without getting rid of the sins that are at the root of the disease. One of the greatest blocks to healing is the sin of unforgiveness. If you embrace unforgiveness, you are following the law of sin. Unforgiveness is one of the spiritual roots of disease. Don't hold on to the wrongs committed by others. Be a doer of the Word. Be a forgiver.

I want to share with you the power of repentance from unforgiveness in the healing of disease. Some years ago, I had

6. Jerry Adler, "Live and Let Live," *Newsweek*, October 3, 2004, https://www.newsweek.com/forgive-and-let-live-129513.

the opportunity to minister to a fifty-year-old pastor's wife who was diagnosed with stage four breast cancer. It had metastasized, and the doctors gave her no hope for survival. She'd been prayed for by her husband and the elders of the church, but there was no change. Her doctor, who was also a member of her church, heard about my work with the spiritual roots of disease and said to her, "Maybe you should call Pastor Wright."

Her husband called me, and then his wife got on the phone. What happened next was a very frank conversation. This dear woman was looking for another prayer for a supernatural healing, but I was looking for the spiritual root of her disease so that she could be healed and set free. I told her, "You have already been prayed for by many. We need to follow the Word of God concerning the law of sin and disease." As we talked about the battle with the law of sin, she began to search her heart. Finally, I asked her, "Do you have any unforgiveness or bitterness against another woman?" Why did I ask that question? Because in my three-decade journey of fighting disease, a high percentage of case histories have revealed that a woman who gets breast cancer has bitterness and unforgiveness in her life, often against another woman.

After my question, this woman became very quiet. Then she admitted, "Yes, I do." I was excited, even though I didn't let it show, because I knew we were moving in the right direction. James 5:16 says, *"Confess your faults one to another, and pray one for another, that ye may be healed."* I knew that her healing required confession, repentance, and forgiveness.

TAKE RESPONSIBILITY FOR YOUR LIFE

I asked this woman what she thought she should do next. "I think I need to repent to the Father." She thought again, and then she said, "Well, I think what I need to do is not just confess to the Father. I need to contact this woman, confess to her that I've had this bitterness, and ask her to forgive me." She would call her to say, "I've had this unforgiveness. I hate it. It is sin in my life. I ask you to forgive me." I knew that when she confessed to the Father and also asked for this woman's forgiveness, she would be forgiven. *"For if ye forgive men their trespasses, your heavenly Father will also forgive you"* (Matthew 6:14). Of course, the Scripture goes on to say, *"But if ye forgive not men their trespasses, neither will your Father forgive your trespasses"* (verse 15). We can't forget that. We must forgive!

Forgiving others is one of the major keys to receiving from God. This pastor's wife made the life-changing decision to take responsibility for her unforgiveness against this other woman. She approached her with a pure heart of conviction to forgive her and to ask for her forgiveness. Even though the cancer was metastasized, I knew the power of the cross would break the power of the enemy over her.

I never heard from her again. However, a few months later, I received a book in the mail entitled *The Biblical Guide to Alternative Medicine*, autographed by the author, Dr. Michael Jacobson. Dr. Jacobson was the woman's medical doctor who attended their church and had counseled her to call me. When I read his book, I discovered that the pastor's wife had received a complete healing from her cancer! God was faithful to His Word!

How did her healing occur? I just brought the truth; she had to be obedient and do the rest. Her heart was opened and submitted to God by confessing and repenting of her sin toward another. She became a doer of the Word and not just a hearer. *"But be ye doers of the word, and not hearers only, deceiving your own selves"* (James 1:22). Why become a doer of the Word? So that we no longer *deceive ourselves*, and we can recover ourselves from the snare of the devil!

WHY WOULD YOU TAKE THEIR SIN?

I have already stated that 20 percent of chronic diseases do not have a spiritual root. However, if you have a disease, wouldn't you want to search the Scriptures and also search your heart? Wouldn't you go to the Lord with this request from Psalm 139, *"Search me, O God, and know my heart: try me, and know my thoughts: and see if there be any wicked way in me, and lead me in the way everlasting"* (Psalm 139:23–24)? When you think of someone in particular, do you feel a high-octane *ping* go off deep inside of you? Consider that you may be holding unforgiveness or resentment in your heart toward that person. If what is keeping you from your healing is the law of sin, which is the opposite of the Word of God, don't you want to repent of it and move on to a life of wholeness and health? Confess it before the Lord and be free.

If you decide to follow the law of sin, instead, and hold a record of wrongs against another person, it will likely produce a disease in your body. That's true even though that person sinned against you—wronged you, betrayed you. It was their sin. But because of your agreement with a spirit of bitterness, you now have a disease.

I need to ask you a very serious question. I don't want you to forget this question as long as you live because your life may depend on it. *Why would you take the sins of another person into your body?*

Jesus took that sin so that you don't have to. He forgave them. He went to the cross, and as He hung there dying, He was asking His Father to forgive the very person that you won't forgive today. If you take another person's failure against you into your heart and into your body, you can expect trouble to come on you in your lifetime. Be kind to yourself and forgive them. Release them, get your heart right with God, and then keep moving on in freedom. You will still have the memory, but God will heal the pain. The kindest thing you can do for yourself is to forgive others.

DON'T BE EASY PICKINGS FOR SATAN!

Feelings can be a source of temptation that comes from Satan's kingdom. That's what happened to Adam and Eve. They had feelings and thoughts. They embraced them. Then, they followed them. Do you think you're not easy pickings for Satan's temptation? Please don't think that you aren't tempted by the law of sin, or that you are stronger than Paul in overcoming temptation! What about Peter? At the Last Supper, Peter basically said to Jesus, "Tonight I will die this death with You." The Lord looked at him over a communion table and answered, "Peter, tonight, you will deny Me three times!" (See, for example, Luke 22:31–34.)

It's clear to see there is a war going on within. God defeated Satan, but Satan still roams this earth like a roaring lion seeking whom he might devour. *"Be sober, be vigilant; because your adversary the devil, as a roaring lion, walketh about, seeking whom he may devour"* (1 Peter 5:8). God desires to free us through His Word and His Holy Spirit, but the enemy wants to capture us through his lies and deceptions. The choice is yours. Who do you want to be your master?

THE POWER OF GRACE AND MERCY

Please don't be discouraged or afraid of the battle we must face between the law of sin and the law of God. God is showing us truth so that He can make us free. *"If the Son therefore shall make you free, ye shall be free indeed"* (John 8:36). When Paul looked at the critical battle in his own life, he cried out, "Who will save me?" His answer is the same as our answer today! *"O wretched man that I am! who shall deliver me from the body of this death? **I thank God through Jesus Christ our Lord**"* (Romans 7:24–25). Our victory in this battle comes from the Lord Jesus Christ!

Jesus's life, death, and resurrection brought us the Father's grace and mercy. God's grace gives us the power to make the right choices. God's grace is teaching us the things we need to know as children of God, and the Holy Spirit is giving us the power to defeat the influence of Satan and the law of sin in our lives. Grace's companion is mercy. Mercy is the amount of time God gives us to figure out what He is saying to us through His

Word and through His Spirit. Thank God that we are living in the dispensation of His grace and mercy!

RESPONDING TO GOD IN LOVE

Through Jesus Christ, God has removed the power of the law and given us the opportunity for our heart to respond to Him, not out of fear, not because of legalism, but because He loves us and we love Him. You can go and sin no more and allow the Lord to renew you in His grace and mercy. It's a daily journey for each of us.

Do not open your life to Satan's lies. Sometimes we fall into his deception and don't even realize it. Keep your spiritual eyes open to the truth of God's Word. You don't have to obey unforgiveness. You don't have to obey anger. You don't have to obey fear. You don't have to obey lust. You don't have to obey shame. You don't have to obey anything that's not God's nature. When having done all to stand, just stand, man or woman of God. Just stand! Let the enemy know your resolve. *"Neither yield ye your members as instruments of unrighteousness unto sin but yield yourselves unto God as those that are alive from the dead and your members as instruments of righteousness unto God"* (Romans 6:13). You must make this decision.

Will you appropriate the freedom the Father has purchased for you through the blood of His Son? Will you choose to embrace the nature and the law of God or the law of sin? Will you choose forgiveness, love, and peace—or will you choose unforgiveness, bitterness, hatred, fear, and anxiety? God has given you a choice. Choose life.

Five

WHO CONTROLS OUR THOUGHTS?

Where do our thoughts come from? Is everything we think from ourselves? For Christians, some of our thoughts are from the Holy Spirit. Some of our thoughts are our own. Some of our thoughts are also from the enemy—Satan. Your body is a *responder* to who you are in thought. It's referred to as the mind-body connection. It's not anything new to a believer. God already told us, *"As a man thinketh in his heart, so is he"* (Proverbs 23:7). God knew what He was talking about! It is a biological truth that the things we think about and dwell on actually become part of who we are. We will never get to the spiritual roots of disease if we don't first understand the biology of how our minds affect our bodies.

This is not a new concept in the medical field, either. Science discovered the mind-body connection long ago. This connection is taught in all medical training centers. What is *not taught* is the *spirit*-mind (soul)-body connection. As a result, not many people understand that it is not just a mind-body connection, but that our spirits are involved as well—it's a *spirit-soul-body* connection.

I'm emphasizing again that you must understand this truth in order to move on to freedom from disease.

We acquire the mind of Christ by meditating on His Word, thinking as He thinks, and embracing God's ways and His nature. We're supposed to be moving forward in God's Word, not shrinking in truth and knowledge. You need to know how to acquire the mind of Christ because your mind plays a crucial role in the spiritual roots of disease. You need to understand that not all of our thoughts come from ourselves. Some of them come from our enemy. And those thoughts bring the roots of disease with them.

THE ORIGIN OF OUR THOUGHTS

We have already established that God is a spirit, the enemy is a spirit, and you are a spirit, with a soul and a body. God communicates with us spirit to spirit. Unfortunately, so does the enemy. You receive thoughts at the spirit level—within you—and record them at the soul level, in your mind and emotions. The important thing to understand about your thoughts is that they might not be yours! They could come from you, from the Holy Spirit, or from Satan's kingdom. That is why it is vital for your health that you understand that your thoughts have different origins.

When a thought passes through our mind, we may naturally assume that it comes from us. However, it might have been given to us by an invisible enemy from an invisible kingdom who will then make it sound just like us by "speaking" in the first person. Satan tempts us with negative thoughts; he plants the thoughts, repeats the thoughts, and we are deceived into accepting them as our own. We embrace them and take ownership of them. Then, the enemy uses those same thoughts to control us spiritually, psychologically, and biologically. Those thoughts are what the Bible calls temptations.

TEMPTATION TRAINS YOU

We are very aware that what the Bible calls temptation, the world has redefined as mere negative emotions or psychological defects. They insist it's just emotional issues rather than a spiritual problem. But that's not what Jesus taught. Jesus taught it was a spiritual problem. Too many Christians are woefully ignorant about temptation. They act like temptation and sin don't exist anymore. The church might dismiss temptation, or they may call it a human problem; some may even go into an altered state of consciousness through prescription drugs to avoid it. But "out of sight, out of mind" is not a spiritual principle! God doesn't want you to be mindless. He wants you to be awake to the truth and to be redeemed from the lies!

Temptation comes to us in thoughts and feelings. Obviously, the thoughts that come to you every day are not always good ones. You might be thinking, "Well, I just wish I wouldn't have these negative, bad thoughts." Unfortunately, none of us is immune to temptation. Not even Jesus was immune to temptation even though He never sinned. You are not immune to the influence of a spirit world that wants to get you to listen. Wake up! You need to understand the Word of God well enough to know what is of God and what isn't. Then you can embrace the truth.

Temptation comes to train you. Be careful what you listen to and what you watch. The enemy wants you to listen to him. He wants to use thoughts and temptations to train you in the law of sin, to train you to be sick. You need to check those thoughts against the Word of God. When the enemy comes to attack you, you need to quit blaming yourself for thoughts that aren't even yours. You've embraced thoughts and feelings like Adam and Eve did. You've been carrying them most of your lifetime. Why do that? Be kind to yourself.

SHORT-TERM AND LONG-TERM MEMORY

Let's look closely at how our mind (soul) is involved in this spirit-soul-body connection. You have an active brain with thoughts popping up all over the place, along with feelings and emotions. Your brain is a miraculous processor for these things. The basics of life depend on your thinking. Your mind is continually dwelling on something—whether good or bad. If you're not meditating on the Word of God, you're meditating on something else.

Initially, what we perceive all around us—what we experience during our day—is stored in our short-term memory. What we have in our short-term memory will be forgotten if it is not moved into our long-term memory. For this to happen, a biological event must take place in our brain called *protein synthesis*. The process, which involves our RNA, is essential for this memory transaction to occur. Once the thought is in long-term memory, we can remember it and recall it. And the more often we recall or dwell on the thought or experience, the more permanent it becomes in our brains.

Listen carefully. After time, *that thought becomes permanently part of your soul.* It becomes a part of your mind, part of your emotions, part of your personality—part *of your biology.* Good thoughts become permanently a part of your biology. The Word of God becomes permanently a part of your biology. And sinful thoughts become a permanent part of your biology, as well. They become part of the way you think and act. For that reason, both God and Satan want their ways to be stored in your long-term memory.

God uses this process that He created in us to build long-term memory when we meditate on His Word, when we meditate on the truths of His love for us. But so does the enemy when we meditate on his lies—things like, "The Bible is outdated; you don't have to follow it." "You're a worthless loser." "You fail at everything you do." You need to hear something six times in order to retain 25 percent of it in your long-term memory. I know that when the enemy comes along, he does not give you a thought only six times. He may give you that thought every day for years on end because he wants to program you to have a disorder or disease. You are in his sights because of a lack of understanding of Satan's devices—his plans and his schemes.

Please understand that this is a journey from the inside out. God wants to influence us from within, by His Spirit and by His Word. The kingdom of darkness wants to influence us from within as well. God speaks to you from within to train you in His nature and righteousness, while the enemy speaks to you from within to train you in death and destruction. Satan has been training the human race in the law of sin since the time of Adam and Eve.

MEDITATE ON GOD'S WORD

In order to allow the Word of God to become a part of your biology, to become flesh of your flesh, you must meditate on it. How often does God say to meditate on the Word? Day and night. *"Blessed is the man that walketh not in the counsel of the ungodly, nor standeth in the way of sinners, nor sitteth in the seat of the scornful. But his delight is in the law of the LORD; and in his law doth he meditate **day and night**"* (Psalm 1:1–2).

God knows that if you meditate on His Word, it will become a permanent part of you. In this way, God has given us *the antidote to the law of sin*. If you do not have this antidote, all you have is the law of sin without the spiritual power to defeat it. You can go on an antidepressant to try to suppress bad thoughts and temptations, but it will not help you change your mindset. What will help you change your mindset is if you read and apply God's Word, which is life and truth, and begin the process of coming out of disease and into freedom! (You can begin to renew your mind while still on the medication. Please do not stop your medicine without the supervision of your doctor.)

Satan is banking on your being so unfamiliar with the truth of God's Word that he can successfully tempt you with the law of sin. He can control your thinking and then blame you, as if the thought behind it were original to you. So, you have the bad thought and the guilt of it, all from his hands. We can be so easily duped by the enemy!

TAKE THOSE THOUGHTS CAPTIVE!

Thankfully, we serve a God of grace and mercy! He is not going to leave us defenseless against Satan's onslaught of thoughts and temptations. Jesus understands our battle against the enemy because He battled him, as well. You know your personal battles. What are you going to do with the thoughts that come from the enemy and compete with the Word of God? You're going to use the spiritual weapons of warfare that God has given you! You're going to take those thoughts captive and cast them down as evil imaginations. *"For the weapons of our warfare are not carnal, but mighty through God to the pulling down of strong holds; **casting down** imaginations, and every high thing that exalteth itself against the knowledge of God, and **bringing into captivity every thought** to the obedience of Christ"* (2 Corinthians 10:5).

What does it mean to "bring every thought into captivity"? It means considering the origin of every thought you have, every feeling, every emotion, every picture, everything that surges through your spirit and mind. Those feelings, apprehensions, and thoughts can cause biological manifestations, such as disease and disorders in your body. You are going to test those thoughts against the Word of God. Are they truth or a trap from the enemy? Then you are going to embrace the truth and not the lie.

Now, I don't want you to think that I am advocating a "mind over matter philosophy." This is not you accomplishing all this in your own strength alone. This is the power of the Word of God and the Holy Spirit enabling you to do what the Word directs you to do! Casting down false imaginations is a powerful weapon that God has given us to fight the enemy. Why would you ignore His help? It's like a soldier going into battle and leaving his rifle behind. Cast down those imaginations and anything that doesn't measure up to the knowledge of God.

Meditating on the Word of God means that you read it, memorize it, think about it often, and embrace it as being truth in your life. You will recognize the source of your thoughts by how they measure against those Scriptures, and you will reject any thoughts that do not line up with God's Word. Take those thoughts captive to the obedience of Jesus Christ and kick them to the curb—for good!

YOU NEED SPIRITUAL DISCERNMENT

When false thoughts come to you claiming that you are not loved by God, or God has rejected you, take hold of those thoughts and ask yourself, "Where did these thoughts come from? Did they originate from the Word of God?" No, they didn't, because God's Word says that if we are believers, God dwells in us and loves us, and nothing shall be able to separate us from His love. *"God is love; and he that dwelleth in love dwelleth in God, and God in him"* (1 John 4:16). *"For I am convinced that neither death nor life, neither angels nor demons...nor anything else in all creation, will be able to separate us from **the love of God** that is in Christ Jesus our Lord"* (Romans 8:38–39).

We all need spiritual discernment. Spiritual discernment requires examining the origin of thought with the guidance of the Holy Spirit. If fear comes to tempt you—whether fear of man, fear of rejection, fear of failure, fear of death, or fear of something else—you can go directly to the Word of God and declare, "That's not from God. According to His Word, God has not given me the spirit of fear! *'God hath not given us the spirit of fear; but of power, and of love, and of a sound mind'* (2 Timothy 1:7). I'm not listening to those lies any longer!" That is how you take hold of those thoughts and cast them down as imaginations!

The lies from the enemy that you once meditated on will become a diminished part of your persona because you're not focusing on them any longer. It will become easier and easier to cast down a lying thought because you recognize what it is, you cast it down, and you move on. That is how you become an overcomer!

No one can do this for you. You must learn to embrace the Word of God for yourself. God will be there to encourage you by His Holy Spirit, but you have to choose to do this. Don't wallow in self-pity or engage in excessive self-talk about your sickness and disease. Don't make excuses. The Holy Spirit lives within you and gives you the strength and the power to make these choices. Take those thoughts captive to the obedience of Jesus Christ. Do it.

RENEWING YOUR MIND

Romans 12:2 says, *"Be not conformed to this world: but be ye transformed by the renewing of your mind."*

The Bible talks about renewing our minds, which is also why God tells us to meditate on His Word day and night. Your mind is renewed, or cleansed, from Satan's lies and thought patterns by being washed with the water of the Word. *"That he might sanctify and cleanse it with the washing of water by the word"* (Ephesians 5:26). This cleansed mind now confronts your bad thinking and teaches you how to think righteously. You can learn how God wants you to think and apply it to your life. If you have fear, anxiety, or stress, this is the process of getting free. This is how we become spiritual people in how we think, speak, and act. I ask God our Father to join you in your journey so that you can be conformed into His image.

As painful as it can be for people to face the truth about hidden things in their lives, at Be in Health, it is our calling to present that truth and compel Christians to face their fears, anxieties, and sins. Don't be afraid. The renewing of our minds must happen for us to have victory. As a result of our minds being renewed in God's Word, we will be delivered from the diseases that afflict the rest of the world. God gave us the key in Romans 12:1–2:

> I beseech you therefore, brethren, by the mercies of God, that ye present your bodies a living sacrifice, holy, acceptable unto God, which is your reasonable service. And be not conformed to this world: but be ye transformed by the renewing of your mind, that ye may prove what is that good, and acceptable, and perfect, will of God.

Listen to God! Do not listen to the world!

Six

THE PATHWAY OF DISEASE

Bless the LORD...who forgiveth all thine iniquities;
who healeth all thy diseases.
—Psalm 103:2–3

I had some personal experiences with the spirit-soul-body connection very early in my ministry. I was a young pastor in my first church. It was a storefront church in Florida, and we were having prayer meetings every Monday night. During one prayer meeting, a young woman came into the church. Her husband was in the car, and he was overcome with muscle spasms, shaking and falling to the floor.

I ran out to the sidewalk and yanked open the passenger door of the car. Her husband was half in the seat and half on the floor, shaking violently. It was so startling that the first thing that came out of my mouth was, "Whoa!" I thought, "What are you going to do with that?" "Call 9-1-1" was the logical answer. But

I stopped first to pray, saying, "Father, I haven't the foggiest idea what's going on, but You do."

I was a pre-med student in college, so I had some knowledge of the human body. One word jumped into my mind as soon as I began praying: *hypothalamus*. I found myself praying this: "I take authority over the spirit of fear that's giving signals to the hypothalamus to produce this involuntary muscle spasm. I command the spirit of fear to be gone, and the hypothalamus to not take any more information from that spirit of fear. Central nervous system, be at peace; muscle spasms, stop now, in Jesus's name." And just like that, it stopped. Her husband sat back up on that passenger seat, and she drove him home. We went back into the prayer meeting in awe of what God had just done.

LAUNCHING A JOURNEY

I was shocked to realize that I had spoken accurately to the evil spirit that had taken over this man's mind with feelings and thoughts that caused him to become fearful. This fear had triggered the hypothalamus gland to begin producing neurological signals causing the involuntary muscle spasms that had him on the floor of his car. I learned a never-forgotten lesson that night: God has given us a connection between the spirit, the soul, and the body.

That night I launched out on a thirty-plus-year journey to study the connection between thought and physiology. The result of those studies are tens of thousands of people worldwide who now have the knowledge for their freedom from disease. It's my desire to pass this knowledge on to you, as well. Some of the details are a little technical, but please keep tracking with me. It is for your life and health.

God has created the human body with a plan for your health. You need to understand how your body is constructed—as well as how that plan is thwarted by the decisions you make in your thought life. God has given you an amazing human body with many highly functioning systems. You have a brain, a nervous system, a cardiovascular system, heart rhythm, skin, hair, eyes, ears, and nose. You have a skeletal form, muscles, kidneys, bone marrow, blood vessels, and lymph glands. You have your liver, lungs, intestines, urinary tract, and endocrine system, including important glands like the amygdalae and hypothalamus glands. This is you. This is what you are on the inside. You are a creative miracle. And all of these systems are highly responsive and regulated by a process that *originates in your brain*.

YOUR BRAIN AND YOUR NERVOUS SYSTEM

There are two parts to your nervous system. First, the *voluntary* nervous system which gives you voluntary control of your body movements. You can tell your arm to rise up and scratch your head when you want to. Second, you have the *involuntary*, or *sympathetic*, nervous system, which God created so that your heart would pump and you could breathe without thinking about it; your digestive organs work, passing food through your body without you giving it another thought. However, if you have a long-term memory full of thoughts that oppose God's Word, your brain can interfere with both the voluntary and the involuntary nervous system, causing them to function improperly; that is what I call the *dis*-ease of function. *Dis*-ease is exactly what it sounds like—the lack of *ease* or health within your spirit and your body's systems.

Now, stay with me here as we go a little further. Look at Chart 1. We are looking at the brain. Your limbic system is the part of the brain that deals with your emotions and your memory. There are four main parts in the limbic system, but to understand the roots of disease, I want to focus on two in particular: the *amygdala* and the *hypothalamus* glands.

Tracking Fear in the Brain

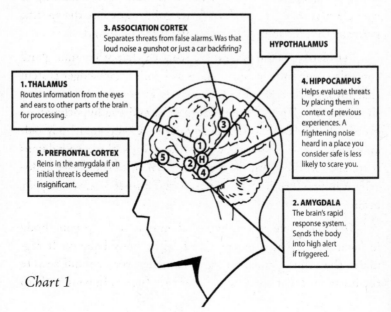

3. ASSOCIATION CORTEX
Separates threats from false alarms. Was that loud noise a gunshot or just a car backfiring?

HYPOTHALAMUS

1. THALAMUS
Routes information from the eyes and ears to other parts of the brain for processing.

4. HIPPOCAMPUS
Helps evaluate threats by placing them in context of previous experiences. A frightening noise heard in a place you consider safe is less likely to scare you.

5. PREFRONTAL CORTEX
Reins in the amygdala if an initial threat is deemed insignificant.

2. AMYGDALA
The brain's rapid response system. Sends the body into high alert if triggered.

Chart 1

The amygdalae are two almond-shaped glands near the frontal lobe area of your brain. Each is a cluster of nerve cells that are responsible for what we call the "fight-or-flight" reaction to emergency situations, stress, and fear. The amygdalae also play a vital role in storing our long-term memories. The amygdalae and the hypothalamus are involved in our deeply felt emotions, whether negative (such as panic, anger, fear) or positive (such as love, laughter, joy).

THE HYPOTHALAMUS: A SMALL GLAND WITH A BIG JOB

How does this affect our bodies in relation to disease? I want to explain to you the importance of the pea-sized gland called the hypothalamus. It's very significant in our understanding of the spiritual roots of disease. We are going to expose the specific pathway that Satan uses to bring disease to mankind.

Let's look at Chart 2 and see what the hypothalamus gland controls. Your endocrine system is a chemical messenger system that involves several important glands in your body, including the pituitary gland, the adrenal glands, and the hypothalamus gland. These glands secrete hormones that keep your body balanced and working smoothly. Of these glands, the *hypothalamus* is considered the brain, or the *control center*, of the entire endocrine system. It is a small but vital gland in the center of your brain.

The main role of the hypothalamus is to keep your body in *homeostasis*, which means in a healthy body balance. It regulates the other glands, telling them when they should secrete the hormones that are necessary *for every system* in your body to

Endocrine System

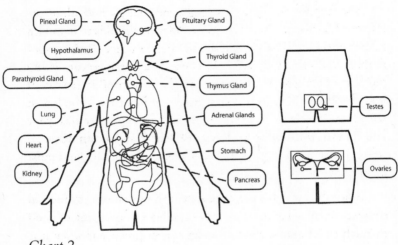

Chart 2

remain in homeostasis, or in a healthy balance. Your body works continually to maintain this balance because without it, you will develop a disorder or disease.

THE MASTER CONTROL

As the master control, the hypothalamus regulates many bodily activities: your body temperature, thirst, appetite and weight control, emotions, sleep cycles, sex drive, childbirth, blood pressure and heart rate, production of digestive juices, and balancing of bodily fluids. It activates your thyroid, which, in turn, affects your metabolism, energy levels, and developmental growth. It stirs the pituitary gland to release the growth hormones we all need.

The hypothalamus is working continually, controlling the release of hormones from the other endocrine glands to maintain homeostasis in all of these systems. For example, if the hypothalamus receives a message that your body temperature is too high, it will trigger the appropriate gland to produce sweat. If it receives the message that your body temperature is too low, it will create heat by shivering. As a result, unless you are sick, your body maintains something close to 98.6 degrees Fahrenheit at all times. It's an astounding amount of work for a small gland most people have never heard of before!

Since the hypothalamus regulates your heart rate, the actual contraction of your heart muscles, and the movement of food through the digestive system, serious problems occur when it is not functioning normally. An interference with the hypothalamus in the function of your cardiovascular system can cause high blood pressure and heart attacks. In the gastrointestinal system, this interference can result in such things as ulcerative colitis, irritable bowel syndrome, diarrhea, vomiting, and nausea.

WHAT YOU MEDITATE ON REGULATES THE HYPOTHALAMUS

Our main focus here is that the hypothalamus is also the center of the spirit-soul-body connection for disease that we have been discussing. This is so important for you to understand. Take a look at Chart 1 again. The cerebral cortex covers the largest part of the brain. It's how we process information, our thinking, language comprehension, problem solving, and—most important for this study—our long-term memory. When you are meditating on thoughts of fear, anxiety, bitterness, anger, self-hatred, or shame, the amygdalae receive and interpret those strong negative emotions and thoughts as a threat. The rest of the limbic system kicks into survival mode, and the hypothalamus gland responds.

The hypothalamus receives these negative messages from your thoughts and may become overwhelmed. The result may be hypo- or hyperactivity in the endocrine system, neurological misfiring in your brain, or neurotransmitter imbalance. Your constant negative thoughts—and the evil spirits behind them—have disrupted the proper working of the hypothalamus gland, and a hypothalamus gland that is not at peace can lead to diseases and disorders in any part of your body.

A lack of homeostasis can affect the gastrointestinal system, create sexual disorders (impotence and frigidity), cause skin diseases (eczema, neurodermatitis, acne, etc.), and lead to diabetes and amenorrhea, fatigue and lethargy, overeating, depression, and insomnia. In addition, it can lead to coronary artery disease, hypertension/disturbance of heart rhythm, tension, headaches, muscle contractions, back aches, rheumatoid arthritis, related inflammatory diseases, asthma, hay fever, and immunosuppressant autoimmune disease. All these conditions stem from a dysfunction with the hypothalamus gland, creating a lack of homeostasis or balance in your body.

Medical science agrees with the role of the hypothalamus in responding to our emotions. Scientists agree that our minds—through strong negative thoughts and emotions—can create an imbalance of homeostasis. As I assured you earlier, I am not an enemy of science. Look at the information it has provided for our understanding of the physical function of the brain and the hypothalamus gland. The medical community has concluded:

> "According to the mind-body or biopsychosocial paradigm, which supersedes the older biomedical model, there is no real division between mind and body because of networks of communication that exist between the brain and neurological, endocrine and immune systems," said Oakley Ray, Professor Emeritus of Psychology, Psychiatry and Pharmacology at Vanderbilt University (Nashville, TN, USA).[7]

Science confirms that there is a direct correspondence between anxiety and palpitations.[8] There is a direct correspondence between hostility and coronary artery thrombosis.[9] There is also a direct connection between shame and irritable bowel syndrome.[10]

---

7. Brower, "Mind-Body Research Moves Toward the Mainstream."
8. Peter Tyrer and David Baldwin, "Generalised Anxiety Disorder," *Lancet* 368 (2006): 2156–66, https://www.sciencedirect.com/science/article/abs/pii/S0140673606698656.
9. Daichi Shimbo et al., "Hostility and Platelet Reactivity in Individuals Without a History of Cardiovascular Disease Events," *Psychosomatic Medicine* 71 (2009): 741–7, https://journals.lww.com/psychosomaticmedicine/Abstract/2009/09000/Hostility_and_Platelet_Reactivity_in_Individuals.7.aspx.
10. Douglas A. Drossman et al., "A Focus Group Assessment of Patient Perspectives on Irritable Bowel Syndrome and Illness Severity," *Digestive Diseases and Sciences* 54 (2009): 1532–41, https://pubmed.ncbi.nlm.nih.gov/19337833/.

THE HYPOTHALAMUS IS THE PATHWAY THE ENEMY USES

Now, how is our spirit-man involved in this connection between the mind, the hypothalamus gland, and disease? Remember, the soul (the mind and emotions) is the bridge between the spirit world and the physical world. God uses the hypothalamus gland to maintain a *balance* of homeostasis in our bodies. The devil uses it to create an *imbalance* of homeostasis. All of this is done through our thoughts and emotions.

If the hypothalamus can be triggered into dysfunction through temptations—and if a lack of homeostasis can cause disease—then the enemy has a clear pathway to bring disease into our lives, doesn't he? The hypothalamus gland is the enemy's entryway to create many diseases in our bodies. Let's walk through this whole process again. Here is the pathway:

Step One: The enemy tempts you with thoughts that oppose the Word of God—thoughts of unrighteousness, such as unforgiveness, bitterness, self-hatred, greed, envy, jealousy, anger, hostility, fear, stress, and anxiety. These are part of the law of sin.

Step Two: If you embrace those unrighteous thoughts and emotions as your own and meditate regularly on them instead of on the Word of God, they become a part of your long-term memory and a part of your actual biology.

Step Three: These elevated negative thoughts and emotions, and the evil spirits behind them, are then communicated from your amygdalae glands and the cerebral cortex to the hypothalamus gland. The hypothalamus then triggers the wrong signals (hormones, etc.) to other vital glands throughout your body.

Now, this isn't a onetime occurrence. It can happen to you day after day, year after year, even beginning in childhood. As a result, your homeostasis becomes unbalanced, and you find yourself combating serious diseases possibly including heart disease, cancer, autoimmune diseases, diabetes, and many more.

For each disease, there is a *door point*, a place where the spirit of infirmity can come in and wreak havoc. The enemy can use thoughts of fear, bitterness, shame, and many other things to wear down the immune system. From that door point, the enemy enters with the spirit of infirmity to bring you disease. *"And he was teaching in one of the synagogues on the sabbath. And, behold, there was a woman which had a spirit of infirmity eighteen years, and was bowed together, and could in no wise lift up herself. And when Jesus saw her, he called her to him, and said unto her, Woman, thou art loosed from thine infirmity. And he laid his hands on her: and immediately she was made straight, and glorified God"* (Luke 13:10–13).

What a devious plan of the enemy! Think about it. The little hypothalamus gland is the only gland that Satan and his spirit of infirmity need to move you in the direction of disease! Instead of our body functioning as God intended, we have *dis*-ease of function. If that *dis*-ease continues, it may transform into a full-blown disorder or disease. Satan understands how the human body functions. The enemy just needs that one gland to set this whole mess in motion. He understands what he needs to do to send you into imbalance and to wreak havoc with your health. He is good at it, but, thankfully, God is so much bigger! That is why we are laying out this knowledge so that you will know how to fight Satan's plan of disease for your life.

I want you to have the victory over the enemy's plan for you! We are intense about this because your life and health are at stake. At Be in Health, we have a God-given zeal to get this message out to as many people as possible. Church, it's time to wake up! Salvation and wholeness are here! I pray for the Holy Spirit to illuminate the minds of everyone reading these pages. I pray that each one may embrace this truth for themselves and their loved ones. We will look now at the specific roots of the autoimmune diseases that you or a loved one need to overcome!

Seven

THE SPIRITUAL ROOTS
OF AUTOIMMUNE DISEASE

I will praise thee; for I am fearfully and
wonderfully made: marvellous are thy works;
and that my soul knoweth right well.
—Psalm 139:14

Our relationship with God is restored when we repent, receive His forgiveness, cast down any thoughts that are not from Him, and renew our minds in His Word. Our relationship with others is restored when we repent, forgive anyone who has wronged us (or ask for forgiveness from anyone we have wronged), and cast aside hatred and malice. But what about the breakdown in our relationship with ourselves? Do you know how many people struggle with self-hatred, self-rejection, and a belief that they are unlovable?

There is a plague in our culture of self-hatred and self-loathing. People devalue their existence, put themselves down, and carry a burden of guilt and shame that is too heavy to bear. It is not from God for His glory, but from the enemy to steal God's glory. "*As he thinketh in his heart, so is he*" (Proverbs 23:7) could never be truer than it is with people who believe that neither God nor anyone else loves them. They are convinced that they are not worthy of that love. Once again, this is the inner workings of our thoughts, believing the enemy's lies to hate ourselves instead of God's Word of love and redemption.

WE ARE ALLERGIC TO OURSELVES

Self-hatred, or what I call an *unloving spirit*, negatively affects the immune system. We have observed this to be especially true in autoimmune diseases because they are closest to mimicking what is really happening spiritually within the person. Oftentimes, the people who hate themselves dwell continually on self-rejecting thoughts and temptations from the enemy. If those thoughts are not cast down, the hypothalamus responds to the temptation and is triggered that something is seriously wrong. Because of the pressure of continuous thoughts of self-hatred and guilt, the hypothalamus begins to misfire and send the wrong impulses to other parts of the endocrine system. The result is that the immune system will weaken and become compromised.

The bottom line of this malfunction? Autoimmune disease. The body becomes allergic to itself! How can this be? Because the person has become allergic to themselves spiritually. Satan's kingdom has persuaded them they are their own worst enemy.

As a result, their immune system is compromised, and the white corpuscles mistakenly identify the antigen markers on the healthy cells in their bodies as a disease or an invader and attacks them. The white corpuscles receive the signal that the healthy tissue is the enemy, and they will either destroy it or produce inflammation.

The body attacks itself if a person attacks himself spiritually in self-rejection, self-hatred, and self-bitterness. The spiritual dynamic that comes into play here is this: the invisible force interfering with the hypothalamus's signal is a spirit of infirmity that redirects the white corpuscles to attack living tissue and to ignore the true invaders, which include bacteria, viruses, and cancers. As the person continues to attack himself or herself spiritually by self-rejection and self-loathing, the body finally responds, and the white corpuscles start attacking the body itself. Quit making yourself the enemy and being allergic to yourself! That is a high price to pay for not loving yourself!

AN UNLOVING SPIRIT

After years of ministry and seeing thousands of individuals diagnosed with an autoimmune disease, I came to the conclusion that most autoimmune diseases are the result of an *unloving spirit* producing feelings of not being loved or accepted, leading to self-rejection, self-hatred, and self-bitterness coupled with guilt. In fact, it could be said that autoimmune diseases are primarily diseases of *self-hatred* with a rider of fear, anxiety, or stress attached. It is a direct biological result of a spirit and soul issue of not accepting who you are, once and for all, in the new birth.

This self-rejection leads to the power of sin that will not let you accept God's righteousness in you. You can't believe the promises of redemption and freedom from God in His Word are for you. You think they only apply to others.

The result is that the spirit-soul-body connection is in play, and the body attacks itself. As we said earlier, there are more than 80 autoimmune diseases or disorders, including multiple sclerosis, rheumatoid arthritis, lupus, Crohn's disease, Graves' disease, psoriasis, diabetes 1, and many more.

The medical community doesn't know the cause or cure for autoimmune disease. Remember, it has an *unknown etiology*. They can't identify the unseen force that causes the body to turn on itself. But we believe that God has revealed an answer to us. The unseen force is the *unloving spirit* that creates self-loathing, self-rejection, guilt, and shame. Science has labeled all auto-immune diseases as incurable. Thankfully, with God, nothing is impossible! We have seen tremendous results in the healing of autoimmune diseases when those afflicted have embrace the truth of these teachings.

WHAT IS SELF-HATRED?

What is self-hatred? It's a temptation from Satan that comes against us in our thoughts to accuse us. According to the Bible, Satan is the one who accuses Christians before God both day and night. *"For the accuser of our brethren is cast down, which accused them before our God day and night"* (Revelation 12:10). When you feel deep, deep feelings of self-accusation, deep, deep feelings of self-loathing, and deep, deep identity rejection, you're actually hearing the voice of that accusing spirit who is accusing you before God.

That's why what we already learned from 2 Corinthians on this subject is so important. *"**Casting down** imaginations, and every high thing that exalteth itself against the knowledge of God, and **bringing into captivity** every thought to the obedience of Christ"* (2 Corinthians 10:5). Hold those thoughts captive to the obedience of Jesus Christ. Don't be ruled by those thoughts and accusations from the enemy. You are to be ruled by the Word of God alone.

Here's what God's Word says about you: you are fearfully and wonderfully made (see Psalm 139:14), and the hand of God is upon you (see 1 Peter 5:6). If you're born again, you're known as a son or daughter of the living God (see 2 Corinthians 6:18). Your name is written in the book of life in heaven (see Philippians 4:3).

Come on! Don't fight against your identity in the Father through Jesus Christ. Embrace it! When you were born again, you became a son or daughter of the Father in heaven. You need a conversion to God's Word! The hand of God is upon you, and you are engraved in the palm of His hands. Read what the Word says about you:

"Behold, I have graven thee upon the palms of my hands" (Isaiah 49:16). *"For the LORD will not cast off his people, neither will he forsake his inheritance"* (Psalm 94:14). *"For he hath said, I will never leave thee, nor forsake thee, so that we may boldly say, The Lord is my helper, and I will not fear what man shall do unto me"* (Hebrews 13:5). You are not rejected by God, so why are you rejecting yourself?

When you hate yourself, it results in self-resentment, self-bitterness, and self-unforgiveness. God forgives you, but you don't think you deserve it, so you won't forgive yourself. Do you realize that you are rejecting Jesus's work for you on the cross? You are telling Him that His death was insufficient to free you from the consequences of sin and whatever you have done wrong. There is a really important issue in our need to be loved. We all need to be loved. Something got in between you and God. You don't feel loved; you feel rejected. Then you become allergic to yourself. A key to this truth: *you may have an identity in the world, and it may even be a successful identity, but you don't have an identity in God.* God is the Author and Sustainer of all that He has made, including us.

Now, let's look at the spiritual roots of several specific autoimmune diseases.

MULTIPLE SCLEROSIS AND IDENTITY REJECTION

According to the National Multiple Sclerosis Society, researchers estimate that nearly one million adults (approximately 913,925) are living with multiple sclerosis (MS) in the United States today. This is more than twice the number reported in previous years based on a national study conducted in 1975 and updates in the following years. About two hundred new cases of MS are diagnosed each week in the U.S., according to the Multiple Sclerosis Discovery Forum. And women are three times more likely to be affected than men.[11]

11. Brandi Koskie, "Multiple Sclerosis Facts, Statistics, and You," Healthline, updated August 21, 2020, https://www.healthline.com/health/multiple-sclerosis/facts-statistics-infographic#Prevalence.

Multiple sclerosis is an autoimmune disease that affects the central nervous system. In the case of MS, for a reason unknown to science, the immune system malfunctions and instead of attacking real invaders, the white corpuscles destroy the fatty substance that coats and protects nerve fibers in the brain and spinal cord. This coating over our nerves is called the myelin sheath. The best way to describe the myelin sheath is to compare it to the insulation coating on electrical wires. Think of a copper wire that is transmitting electricity. That wire is covered with insulation to protect people from being shocked and to protect the wire from being destroyed. Our nerves are created in a similar way. We have a myelin sheath encasing every nerve to protect us from nerve pain and to protect the nerve from damage.

With multiple sclerosis, the white corpuscles mistakenly recognize an antigen marker for a foreign invader on the myelin sheath. The white corpuscles take a "bite" out of the myelin sheath to destroy it. That is called a *sclerosis*. *Multiple* sclerosis is multiple bites of the myelin sheath around multiple nerves. The white corpuscles can sever the nerve itself once the myelin sheath has been destroyed, and nerve damage can become progressively worse. In some cases, the limbs lose all their mobility, resulting in the need for a wheelchair.

I have found through decades of research and case histories that multiple sclerosis is deeply rooted in self-hatred. The afflicted person may ask such questions as "Why am I here?" "Who am I?" "Who cares?" This goes beyond an identity problem to *total rejection* of one's identity. The spiritual root cause of multiple sclerosis is a deep, deep root of self-hatred.

WHO AM I? CONFERENCE

I did a conference a couple of years ago called *Who Am I?* and I discussed three very important questions: (1) Who am I?; (2) Why am I here?; and (3) Who cares? These are the battles I see even with Christians. We have an orphan's mentality. Some of us feel fatherless, and we are desperately searching for meaning in our lives. Who cares? The Father cares! Your acceptance of His love can defeat autoimmune disorders in your life.

A self-rejection disease, such as multiple sclerosis, occurs when you do not accept who you are in creation. Something may have happened in your life for which you have never forgiven yourself. Guilt and shame have followed you through the years. You're always looking over your shoulder for somebody else's approval and not getting it. Some of you are living in families that do not know how to love each other. Others may have families full of people like Job's friends—they act like they are there for you, but they're really accusing you. But you have a true Father. You have THE Father. Don't embrace the principles of death. Stop it. Embrace the principles of life found in the Word of God for your own sake.

HEALED OF MULTIPLE SCLEROSIS

At Be in Health, we have rejoiced for years with a woman named Dana who has a miraculous testimony of God's healing power over multiple sclerosis.

"I'm always amazed when thinking about how God delivered and healed me. Especially that He did this when I wasn't seeking it and didn't even know to seek it. It is an amazing mercy of God.

"I was diagnosed with multiple sclerosis (MS) in October of 2008. I was exhibiting signs of a neurological disease that was progressing quickly, starting with restless leg, loss of control of my left side, and my hand and feet curling inward. When my family doctor saw me, he ordered an emergency MRI, which revealed lesions on my brain and a 4.5-mm lesion on my spinal cord in my neck. An immediate follow-up exam with a neurologist revealed places all over my body where I had no feeling. His prognosis was devastating! It included a future of blindness and the use of a wheelchair. He ordered five days of prednisone delivered intravenously, starting that night in the hospital emergency room. The prednisone did help me recover much of what I had lost in the week leading to the diagnosis. With the Lord's help, I was able to manage the disease for the time I had it and avoid blindness and wheelchairs and all the worst news of my initial diagnosis.

"But God was working on something so much better than disease management for me, and I did not know it because my story of healing doesn't begin with me. It came through my sister, who is a missionary in Africa, and her journey seeking the Lord for answers to both her health and her spiritual issues. In her own crises, the Lord led her to Dr. Wright's book *A More Excellent Way* and to attend one of his conferences in South Africa. She was healed of severe asthma and much else, attended a For My Life retreat in the States, and came to live near us for the final months of their home sabbatical! Praise God! During her time at home, my sister was on a mission to share the truth of healing with her family; we were her primary mission field! We all were sick with various diseases. Our dad was a pastor, but we didn't know we needed the Physician!

"I was astounded at the change in my sister and very intrigued to know what had brought it about. Late in the evening, on July 4, 2011, when everyone else had gone to bed, she began telling me of her time at For My Life and that she had witnessed ministry to a woman with MS. We were standing at the time, as she was telling me the story of this woman's life. At one point, she described how the woman cried, 'I will never forgive myself for....' As soon as she spoke those words, my vision began to narrow, and I felt ready to faint. I interrupted my sister because I needed to sit down or I might fall down. This came from nowhere, and I'd never had anything like it happen before.

"While we sat, she started asking me questions about whether I had a lot of fear in my life or unforgiveness, but I struggled to listen. I was puzzling over what had just happened to me and why I had almost fainted. Suddenly, my sister surprised us both by asking, "What about that babysitter, Gerry?" Gerry was a teenage girl who babysat my siblings and me when we were young—I was six years old, my sister was four, and my brother was two. She was hurting my younger siblings, and I felt responsible because I was the oldest and hadn't told our mother. I answered her, 'I will never forgive myself for not protecting you and our brother. And I am evil because I know that I am uncovered and am a coward.'

"At that moment, my sister spoke words that went straight into my heart. She explained that, for years, a spirit of guilt had taught me the lies that I was guilty and evil, but that God had made provision for guilt. I was to confess it to Him, and He would forgive me and cleanse me from all unrighteousness. In love, my sister assured me that I am not evil, that God did not make me evil, but that another evil spirit had joined with guilt and taught me I was evil.

"I never believed a Christian could be affected so strongly by evil spirits, but I understood these words were truth, and I received them in my heart. I began to weep as she shared Psalm 139 with me, and also the truth that Jesus would have died for me even if I was the only one. Her words washed over me and flowed straight to my heart. When she suggested I confess these things to God in prayer, I was ready! After I repented, she cast out a spirit of guilt and a spirit of self-hatred. And I felt so NEW, completely NEW!

"When I crawled into bed next to my husband, who immediately put his arm around me, I received that embrace like I had never received it before. Even that was completely new. As I shared with him what had just happened to me, I realized that it mirrored the story of the other woman with MS whose words matched mine: 'I will never forgive myself for....'

"I had been blinded to so much: what sin looked like, confessing my guilt and shame, my need for deliverance—and my journey was only beginning. I dedicated myself to learning more and seeking out what else I might need to confess before my forgiving Father. My prayer life changed dramatically—I had never been able to pray to my heavenly Father, only addressing Jesus in my prayers—even though I knew it was more biblical to address the Father. It wasn't until I finally got my own copy of *A More Excellent Way* that I realized that I could expect physical healing as a result of my repentance. As I read, whenever the Holy Spirit revealed something I needed to confess, I would close the book, acknowledge it to God, receive forgiveness—sometimes rebuking a spirit—then continue reading. And it didn't stay between me and God only; there were people I needed to ask for forgiveness, even from the past. I understood what sin really looked like—I drank it all up as from a fire hose—and I was being changed! In the course of time, I realized I had no more MS symptoms! I waited until I had none for a month before I shared with anyone my belief that I was healed from multiple sclerosis!

"A decade has passed since that blessed July Fourth night when God interrupted the course of my life and set me on a completely different path. I have no MS symptoms. I am healed, delivered, and a new creature in the Father's love!"

—Dana S.

Eight

RHEUMATOID ARTHRITIS AND LUPUS

RHEUMATOID ARTHRITIS AND SELF-ACCUSATION

Rheumatoid arthritis is a disfiguring autoimmune disease. The white corpuscles are influenced by a spirit once again and misidentify the antigen markers on the connective cartilage of the joints. They say to that cartilage, "You are the enemy!" Once again, the white corpuscles attack the body by destroying the body's connective cartilage and inflammation occurs.

Anything that relates to the skeleton or bones has an *identity problem* as the spiritual root. Individuals with rheumatoid arthritis suffer from self-accusation and can't help comparing themselves with others. They don't accept themselves as they are. They think that they are inferior to others, and, as a result, they become allergic to themselves. They have a very negative way of viewing themselves, the world, and God. We need to understand that we are meant to be unique individuals and not clones of one another. We are fearfully and wonderfully made. We are not made in the image of another human; we are made in the image of God.

The saddest part of rheumatoid arthritis is that those who have it believe that they are not as good as everyone else. Then, as their joints lose flexibility, parts of their body become deformed, resulting in misshapen fingers and bent legs. In the end, these individuals look worse and feel worse about themselves. It is crucial that they repent of their negative self-projections and begin to find their identity in the Father through Jesus Christ.

Sandy is a woman who had been diagnosed with rheumatoid arthritis (RA). For a number of years, she suffered a great deal of pain in her joints. Sandy loved cooking for her family. Once she became sick, she couldn't shop for the food; she couldn't prepare it; she couldn't cook it any longer. Because of her RA, she could barely walk; she used a handicap parking tag on her car for years. She was on a horrible journey because the enemy had programmed her against herself.

Sandy and her husband, Phil, decided to attend a For My Life retreat to learn how she could receive healing and wholeness. They were both convicted as they heard the truth of the spiritual roots of disease. Sandy searched her heart before the Lord and discovered that she had accepted lying thoughts of self-hatred and self-rejection for many years. The enemy had held her captive with his lies. Sandy repented of accepting those lying thoughts and embraced the truth of the Father's love for her through the sacrifice of His Son Jesus. She was renewed in His love and freely accepted His forgiveness. After returning home from For My Life, Sandy never needed to use that handicap parking tag again!

She had been healed and set free by receiving God's truth about her identity in her Creator.

Today, Sandy no longer has rheumatoid arthritis. Her pain is gone, and she is enjoying eight-mile bike rides on the beach with her husband of thirty-seven years. She says that her life is actually better now than before she had the RA. She is a free woman because she rejected the enemy's lies and received her forgiveness in Jesus Christ. Her identity in the Father has been restored.

LUPUS AND GUILT

Your organs are the core of your biology. Lupus is an autoimmune disease where the white corpuscles mistakenly target the antigen marker on the connective tissue of the organs. As the white corpuscles begin to destroy the connective tissue around the organs, they produce symptoms such as pain, fatigue, fever, shortness of breath, and others. In lupus, the primary trigger point or spiritual root is *guilt*. Because of something, or perhaps many things, in life, the individual refuses to forgive themselves and carries deep guilt. Lupus is diagnosed more often in women than in men.

Guilt is a powerful force against us. It is essential that we understand the devices Satan uses to bring the spirit of infirmity into our midst. To thwart Satan's plans, we must forgive ourselves and let the guilt go. Guilt defies a risen Christ and forgiveness. Guilt is an anti-Christ spirit. Guilt doesn't come from God! In Psalm 103:12, we discover that God has separated us from our sins as far as possible: *"As far as the east is from the west, so far hath he removed our transgressions from us.*" How much further than that can God separate you from your sins? Why would you embrace guilt for the thing that God has forgiven you for? Why hang on to things in your personality that don't come from God?

In the medical world, lupus is considered incurable, but I have been blessed to see many people healed of this autoimmune disease, including Lauren, whose testimony is below.

"Shortly after graduating from college in 2007, I married my boyfriend. After just a year and a half of marriage, I decided I had made a mistake. I moved into my own apartment and filed for divorce. He was not a bad guy, but I decided he was not right for me. My actions were selfish, and I began to feel a great deal of guilt for divorcing him. I received hate mail from my ex-in-laws, who said horrible things about me. The guilt continued to grow deeper for about three years before I started to experience strange symptoms and went to see a doctor.

"When I was diagnosed with lupus, the doctor told me that there was no cure—all they could do was 'manage' the disease. I walked out of the office and called my sister while I was still standing in the hallway. She told me immediately about Be in Health and soon after gave me a copy of Dr. Wright's book *A More Excellent Way*. The spiritual roots described in the book were so accurate that I was shocked! The book was talking directly to me. I saw that guilt was the root of lupus in my life, and I knew that I had to make a major change. I attended a three-day conference that Dr. Wright held in Minnesota, and I hung on to every word he said. I was blown away by the truth that I heard!

"I needed to learn how to accept God's forgiveness and how to forgive myself. Growing up, I thought that you asked for forgiveness and then hoped for the best. Through what I learned at Be in Health, I realized I could ask for forgiveness and truly receive it. My sins were *truly* forgiven because of what Jesus did at the cross. I had to forgive myself, as well, which took some time, but I was able to do it.

"My healing from lupus wasn't instantaneous; it was a process. In the beginning, I begged God to heal me from the lupus symptoms instantaneously. But later, I realized that He was working on something so much greater. He was teaching me slowly and bringing me closer to Him because He wanted me to stay close to Him permanently. God was not only interested in my physical healing but in the recovery of my spirit, as well!

"As I share this now, guilt and shame are defeated in my life. I feel no guilt or shame about the divorce because I have confessed it as a sin to God and asked for and received His forgiveness! In 2014, I attended a one-week For My Life retreat and was water baptized. After that week, my symptoms gradually disappeared! It was not an easy process, and it took time and lots of learning, but I can say with confidence that I am now healed from lupus.

"Today, I am happily married to my second husband. When I was diagnosed with lupus, the doctor told me that because of the harsh medication, I shouldn't even try to get pregnant. Since I've been healed and no longer need that medication, we have had two sons. During my pregnancy with my second son, the doctors still considered me high risk because of my health history. But at each of my weekly ultrasounds, they saw great results, and my son was born totally healthy and strong! I am so grateful to Be in Health for sharing the truth with me. And so grateful to God for His healing promises! I pray that my testimony will help others overcome, as well!"

—Lauren H.

SEVEN THINGS I PRACTICED TO HELP ME OVERCOME LUPUS:

+ I asked for and received forgiveness from God, because Jesus died for my sins on the cross. I reminded myself of that daily.

+ I did not identify with the disease; I always referred to it as *the* lupus, never *my* or *mine* because it was just something that was currently affecting me.

+ I kept my confidence in God, knowing that He was going to heal me, and believing in Him and His timing for my healing.

+ I read the testimonies of others' healing. I remained hopeful always, even when it seemed impossible.

+ I daily submitted to God and resisted the devil. I belonged to God, and the devil no longer had any rights to my life.

+ I immediately rebuked guilty thoughts that would pop into my head. In fact, I would turn it around and say, "Good thing I am forgiven! Thank You, God!"

+ I thanked God continually for the healing that I knew was coming. Of course, now I continue to thank God often for my healing and all my other blessings.

Nine

CROHN'S DISEASE AND GRAVES' DISEASE

CROHN'S DISEASE AND PERFORMANCE DISORDER

Crohn's disease is an autoimmune disease where the neurotransmitters are once again giving a false signal to the white corpuscles. In this situation, the white corpuscles decide that the antigen marker for an invader is on the lining of the colon and often into the small intestine. As they begin to "eat" the intestinal lining, they produce inflammation, ulceration, bleeding, and pain. It is a serious disease. Don't forget that the medical world does not know why a malfunction occurs that signals for the white corpuscles to attack the body. We know that the enemy is working to weaken the immune system until the spirit of infirmity can come in and rule in our bodies.

In studying case history after case history, I've come to the conclusion that Crohn's disease is a *performance disorder* where the individual is extremely driven to do everything right in order to keep the people around him happy. There is also guilt involved with Crohn's disease because those who have it believe that they are not capable of doing anything right. Those suffering with Crohn's disease become a false burden bearer of others. They pick up other people's issues and blame themselves if things don't go right for others. They blame themselves for other people's unhappiness, as if they were responsible for others' failures as well as their own. So much revolves around the importance of performance.

The person with Crohn's disease can even hyperventilate in fear that there might be a problem going on even when there is no problem. It's a constant, constant self-conflict issue surrounding performance. The answer to your healing from Crohn's disease is to repent from trying to please man, from taking on too many of the burdens of others and from carrying their guilt for the things that they don't do right. Those with Crohn's disease must embrace the love and acceptance that the Father has for them.

GRAVES' DISEASE AND THE THYROID

Graves' disease is an autoimmune disease where the white corpuscles are congregating together in the thyroid. This produces a swelling and inflammation that causes the thyroid to overproduce the hormone thyroxin. This condition is also called hyperthyroidism. With Graves' disease, you experience excessive fatigue, severe heart palpitations, a developing goiter, and bulging eyes. Graves' disease usually appears in females and, if left untreated, can be life-threatening.

The spiritual root behind Graves' disease is a performance disorder similar to Crohn's disease, even though it attacks a completely different part of the body. Medical science's answer to Graves' disease is to use radioactive chemicals to destroy the thyroid, and then put you on thyroid medicine for the rest of your life. God's prescription is that you be healed of the underlying roots that are causing the disease, and live in health.

We have a family friend, whom I will call Jeanine, who called me several years ago after she was diagnosed with Graves' disease. She had been aware of my teachings for several years and wanted to talk to me about the spiritual roots involved. I answered her, "I know a little bit about autoimmune disease, and I know about you. Jeanine, you just care too much. You have a performance disorder.

"You've got all these people coming to your house; you teach them, and you try to get them well. They won't listen to you. They won't do the first principles, but they keep coming back, and you are taking on their failures as if they were your own. Admit it; they are wearing you out. They're calling you and wanting prayer, but they won't do what the prayer represents. You feel responsible for them, and now you feel like you failed them." In tears, her response was, "You know me too well."

Jeanine began to go to God to change her heart and mind, confessing her sins of taking on the burdens of other people's lives. She prayed and began to meditate on the Word daily from a sincere heart. She took those thoughts of guilt and self-accusation captive to the obedience of Jesus Christ, casting them down because they were not from God but from the enemy. In time, she returned to her doctor who did a blood test and then gave her good news: "Your thyroid is functioning normally. There are no more signs of Graves' disease!" All autoimmune activity had stopped. Jeanine is alive and well today because she applied God's truth.

RESTORED TO THE FATHER

We have seen Graves' disease healed in a number of people over the years whose lives were restored by the biblical truth of repentance of performance disorder and acceptance of the Father's love. This is another woman's amazing testimony of being set free from disease, along with her family members.

"My first visit to Thomaston, Georgia, for the For My Life retreat was several years ago. My life was in shambles; it had become unrecognizable to me. I knew I needed help, but I had no idea which direction to turn. My life and my marriage had been spiraling downward for several years. A secret life of pornography and infidelity that I knew absolutely nothing about had been exposed. My heart started beating unusually fast as one of the many side effects of stress and anxiety. I had been leaning excessively hard on alcohol, and it had become an addiction.

"After six months with an uncontrollable heart rate, I was diagnosed with severe Graves' disease and hyperthyroidism. My pulse stayed at a steady 125 to 130 beats per minute! I was in a constant state of near panic attack, and my heart felt as if it was bruising the inside of my ribs, especially when I lay down to rest. I also had paralyzing pain across my back, down my left arm, and into my pinky that mimicked a heart attack. It became so bad at times that the only thing I could do was get into a fetal position to try to make it stop. Graves' disease had affected my eyes, as well, with my left eye bulging out of its socket. After going on thyroid medicine to counteract the symptoms, I gained twenty pounds, which did not help my already zero self-confidence. I was a mess.

"I had heard of the For My Life retreat, but I was really afraid they might not accept me, that my symptoms were too extreme for them. A dear friend agreed to go with me; so, instead of celebrating our fiftieth birthdays together, we drove from South Florida to Georgia. We arrived on Saturday night at the campground and attended church the next morning. After service, we stayed behind so I could speak with Dr. Wright. My friend spoke for me, as I was extremely anxiety ridden at the time. Dr. Wright's only comment to me was said with much love: "You're just a girl." At the time, it didn't make much sense, but as the week went on, I grew to understand the deeper meaning behind it. It was his kind way of saying that it wasn't my responsibility to try to fix the whole world. It was a release for me, knowing that I did not have to perform beyond my ability.

"In the very first day, I learned that naming 'my diagnosis' was claiming or accepting 'my disease.' The words that came out of my mouth were more powerful than I realized. *'Death and life are in the power of the tongue: and they that love it shall eat the fruit thereof'* (Proverbs 18:21). The evil spirits that I had been in agreement with were running and ruining my life; and, yes, I was just a girl. I thought I understood Christianity. I thought I had a basic idea of what the Word meant in my life. I realized I was such a spiritual baby, and I had so much growing up to do.

"The week uncovered so much wisdom and truth that my mind was reeling. The enemy tried his best to keep me from receiving what God had planned for me. Wednesday night, while doing homework, I started to feel like I was really having a heart attack. I tried my best to breathe through the symptoms, slowing my pulse a bit and thinking about everything that I had learned so far that week. I realized this was just a ploy of the spirit of fear. I had fallen for that trick one too many times. After recognizing and rebuking that spirit, I made it through that night and slept like a baby.

"Thursday was baptism at the end of the day. I have no words to describe the feelings that were pulsing through me by now. I felt for the first time that I had the knowledge to pray the symptoms away and walk in peace. Baptism was a phenomenal expression of that understanding for me. Friday closed out the week with empowering prayers and the rebuking of spirits over every part of our body, followed by individual prayer. I left that week with such a fortune in my spiritual bank account, I felt like I could *walk on water*! I had heard of many miracles that had taken place that week, but the biggest miracle to me was inside 'the girl' who had arrived six days earlier. I had an internal change. I felt a confidence that only the Lord, His truth, and His love can give. I was made new.

"The miracles in my family continued. I returned to For My Life with my two daughters, one of whom was struggling with deep-seated fears and suicide ideation at the time. The counselor we had been seeing was pushing an inpatient program for psychiatric care. I found myself slipping into fear for my daughter but remembered the teachings from my weeks at Be in Health; we packed our car and headed to Thomaston. My struggling daughter was impacted with such love and freedom after one week that she asked if we could stay for a second week so she could attend the retreat a second time! God had transformed her heart and mind as she opened herself to receive His healing love. Her life began again that week—a new life, a life of freedom. Both of my daughters have applied these biblical truths to every aspect of their lives. What a great gift as a mom, to see her children walking in truth.

"A final family blessing was when my husband and I decided to attend together. It was an incredible bonding time. We will never be the same as a couple. What the enemy had planned for destruction, God blessed to His perfection. I now feel cherished and loved by my husband, and he knows I love and respect him in a godly way that builds him up as a man of God. What I thought was lost has not only been resurrected, but our marriage is better than ever.

"Oh, and by the way, that medical diagnosis I used to claim as mine? It is no longer a part of my story! My negative blood work and all symptoms and side effects of Graves' disease have long been gone, I no longer turn to alcohol for help, my eye is back to normal, and my life is beyond blessed. Thank You, good, good Father, for showing me the way to peace and true joy through Your truth."

—Donna B.

Ten

DIABETES 1, PSORIASIS, AND MORE

Diabetes 1 is an autoimmune disease where the pancreas no longer produces the insulin needed to control the sugar level in the body. The body's own immune system—which was created to fight harmful bacteria and viruses—mistakenly identifies the antigen markers on the pancreatic islets and attacks and "eats" them. As a result, the pancreas islets are destroyed and can no longer produce the insulin needed to move sugar (glucose) into the cells, and the sugar builds up in the bloodstream. This can lead to life-threatening conditions.

Although adults can still develop type 1 diabetes, it usually starts in childhood and is a direct result of living in a hostile or unloving family environment, particularly with rejection from a father. A child may begin to think, "Something is wrong with me." He attacks himself in his mind and with his mouth; the result is that the body attacks the body. An unloving spirit is at the root of type 1 diabetes. It can be inherited because an unloving spirit can track down through the generations and bring an unloving spirit into a child's life.

We have seen many people healed of diabetes. There has to be an absolute change in people that allows them to receive the love of God in order for healing to happen. (Please do not stop taking your insulin until your doctor has confirmed that you no longer have diabetes.)

One side note: This book is covering autoimmune diseases, which include type 1 diabetes. Type 2 diabetes is an anxiety/stress disorder where the white corpuscles interfere with the function of the pancreatic tissue, but the islets are not destroyed; they are simply not functioning properly. The possible spiritual roots of type 2 diabetes are many, including fear of failure, fear of man, drivenness, and an inability to receive love. Type 2 diabetes and stress disorders are covered in more detail in my books *A More Excellent Way*, *Exposing the Spiritual Roots of Disease*, and *Exposing the Spiritual Roots of Diabetes*, all published by Whitaker House.

PSORIASIS

Psoriasis is an autoimmune disorder in which the white corpuscles receive a misfiring from the brain and begin congregating on the skin. Normally, our skin cells die and flake off of our skin, but with the inflammation caused by autoimmune disease, the dead cells build up on the skin instead, creating scaling, flaking, redness, and hardness. It can be an itchy and painful disease that has no known cause or cure; health care professionals prescribe ointments and therapies for disease management. In our years of experience, we have seen that psoriasis is spiritually rooted in self-hatred, lack of self-esteem, and conflict with identity.

Jake and Penny are a couple who shared their testimony of gaining victory over many illnesses, including psoriasis. Here is their testimony.

Penny began, "We had never heard of the ministry of Be in Health before, but one day we found videos of their teachings on YouTube. Our journey to a healthy life began by watching their mini teachings on the spiritual roots of disease. We would watch a session, search our hearts, and then ask the Lord to forgive us for not loving ourselves, to forgive us for believing the lies of the enemy, and for not finding our identity in Him.

"Jake had been struggling with psoriasis for a number of years; it was a quarter-inch thick, red and scaly from the elbow to his hand on both arms. While watching the Be in Health mini-series on psoriasis, we learned that it was an autoimmune disease as a result of not loving yourself. We began putting into practice the teachings of repentance to God for believing the lies of the enemy and embracing the love of the Father."

Jake added, "Daily, I was embracing the Word of God and loving on myself the way God intended." Penny continued, "One hot summer day, we were watching TV at our home in Texas when I glanced over at Jake, who was wearing a short-sleeved shirt. I looked again and exclaimed, 'Your psoriasis is disappearing!' The psoriasis had shrunk considerably on both his arms and his calf. We were so excited, and our faith began to really grow. Today, months later, his psoriasis is gone completely. He's no longer up at night scratching. Jake had been healed of an autoimmune disease. But it didn't end there.

"We also watched sessions on the healing of PTSD, type two diabetes, and sleep apnea, all areas that Jake had struggled with for years. All of these diseases and disorders were gone from his life as we applied the teachings on restoring our identity in the Father and rebuking the spirit of infirmity that was harassing his life."

Jake added, "I've been relieved of all of this stuff that I'd been carrying for years and years. I wasn't even aware of it, but it had been piling up decade by decade, experience by experience. Now, I'm free, and I feel literally thirty pounds lighter!"

Penny ended the interview, her voice cracking with emotion. "When we got saved, we got the part of the story of what we needed to do to get into heaven. Through these teachings, we have learned what we need to do to live successfully and in health here on earth. We're not victims anymore. We can rise up and be the man and woman of God that He created us to be. And we are so very grateful for that!"

HEALING FROM INTERSTITIAL CYSTITIS AND SARCOIDOSIS

Interstitial cystitis (IC) is an autoimmune disease where the white corpuscles attack the bladder, causing bladder pressure and pain, often accompanied by pelvic pain. Symptoms usually begin with an increase in urinary frequency and urgency. A significant majority of those diagnosed with IC are women who experience symptoms that range from mild discomfort to severe, debilitating pain. For the more severe cases, which include ulcers on the bladder wall, this disease can have a devastating effect on lifestyle and day-to-day activities.[12]

12. "What Is Interstitial Cystitis?" Interstitial Cystitis Association, https://www.ichelp.org/about-ic/what-is-interstitial-cystitis/.

Interstitial cystitis has similar symptoms to bladder infections, but there is no bacteria involved. Once again, the body is attacking itself. The white corpuscles have received a misfiring from the brain; mistaking the antigen markers on the bladder lining for an invader, they begin to attack. In severe cases, the bladder lining is covered with red, bleeding ulcers. Medical treatments are varied from simple stress relieving activities all the way to aggressive painkillers.[13]

The spiritual roots of interstitial cystitis are self-hatred, guilt, and shame. The immune system has been weakened by the enemy, and the spirit of infirmity has taken hold. The white corpuscles begin attacking the lining of the bladder to bring destruction and disease. But the Father, who wants you to live in health, brings life, as you will see below in the history of Janice L., who struggled with both interstitial cystitis and sarcoidosis, among other diseases, and was set free.

Sarcoidosis is a rare inflammatory autoimmune disease that causes small patches of red and swollen tissue (called granulomas) to develop in different organs in the body. It can develop in any organ, but most of the time, the white corpuscles mistakenly attack the lungs and the skin, causing inflammation. The symptoms of sarcoidosis typically include fatigue, shortness of breath, a persistent cough, and tender, red bumps on the skin. Since medical science has no known cure, the goal is to manage the disease with medicine to bring it into remission. By God's grace, once the self-hatred and unloving spirit behind this disease have been dealt

---

13. "What Is Interstitial Cystitis?" Interstitial Cystitis Association.

with, and their identity in the Father has been restored, individuals can be healed from this disease.

JANICE'S HEALING TESTIMONY

"As a young mother at just twenty-six years old, I began a painful journey of disease. First came the diagnosis of sarcoidosis, an interconnective tissue disease that attacks your organs. It attacked my lungs, and the doctors had to biopsy my liver and spine, as well. I lost a lot of weight, was very weak and tired, and had breathing issues. In the years following, I was hit with one autoimmune diagnosis after the other—interstitial cystitis, lichen sclerosis, hypoglycemia—and they were all considered incurable.

"I carried these illnesses, along with others, throughout my young adult years, managing them as best I could with medical help, until I was in my early fifties and my daughter gave me Dr. Henry Wright's book *A More Excellent Way*. I started reading it and was amazed that it was filled with answers of hope for me. The thing that stood out to me the most, though, was something I had a hard time wrapping my head around. I had been a Christian for years, but I had never heard about the devastating results that self-hatred and self-loathing can do to our bodies. My husband and I, along with our daughter, made an appointment to see Dr. Wright when he was speaking at a conference in Sarasota, Florida. That was my first giant step toward wholeness—spirit, soul, and body.

"The following year, my husband and I attended a For My Life retreat and learned about the spiritual roots of autoimmune disease, and so many other things that affect us when we accept the lies of the enemy instead of embracing the truth of God's Word. I hadn't realized how important this was to our health and wholeness. I began to apply so many things to my life that I had never been taught in church—about the Father's love for me, and how important it is for me to love myself.

"In addition to the autoimmune diseases, I also suffered with fibromyalgia, a stress disorder that brings pain in your muscles and ligaments, fatigue, and insomnia. I learned that the spiritual root of fibromyalgia was from carrying so much fear and anxiety because of a father who wasn't really present for me, and then from my husband who was very driven. The spirits of fear, drivenness to perform to earn love, and guilt—I took it all on as I believed the enemy's lies. At For My Life, I learned how important it was to be easy on myself and not be driven to perform for those around me.

"I believe that the prayers of deliverance over my life were also vital. I was delivered of the spirits of self-hatred, self-resentment, self-bitterness, fear, and rejection. I know that was a key to my healing and recovery. I've also been delivered from the spirit of death and the spirit of infirmity. The enemy was after me. He stole from me for over twenty-five years of my life, but God is the great restorer!

"Praise God, after the For My Life retreat, I was set free of the fibromyalgia almost immediately. Being healed from the autoimmune diseases didn't happen as quickly. It took three or four more years before my healing was complete with all my symptoms gone. Since I had dwelt on the enemy's lies of self-hate for over twenty-five years, I needed to meditate on God's Word and allow it to transform how I felt about myself, to transform how I understood God's love for me.

"I read Psalm 139 regularly, that I was fearfully and wonderfully made. I studied Psalm 103:3, that God forgives all of my sins and heals all of my diseases. Well, if I believe that God forgives all my sins, why don't I believe He can heal all my diseases? I began to believe that He could. I also meditated on Jesus's command that I must not only love God with all of me, but that I must love myself. (See Mark 12:30–31.) I finally understood that God's perfect will is not just to heal me but to keep me walking in health. And during that time, every one of those autoimmune symptoms disappeared. I was healed and free!

"I've been in the church since I was in my twenties. I was prayed for and anointed with oil many times, but I was not healed until I started believing and applying the Word of God. Jesus is my healer. I had to believe that. When we went to For My Life, I saw it modeled before me, and I realized it was truth. It increased my faith that there's more to God and His plans than I knew. I wanted to know the more.

"Today, over fifteen years since the last symptom disappeared, I am still free of all of it. I'm seventy-one, and I have more energy than I did when I was a young mother. I had a lot of brain fog back then, which is completely gone. My ability to function in every way is mine. I've got my life back. Free from all of it. My husband and I have been pastoring a church for the last fourteen years, where we share the power of the Word of God, including how He makes us whole—spirit, soul, and body!"

—Janice L.

THE ANTIDOTE TO AUTOIMMUNE DISEASE

I want you to hear my heart for your health and freedom from autoimmune diseases. Even if the autoimmune disease you have been diagnosed with isn't listed in this book, all autoimmune diseases are an issue of self-hatred and self-conflict. I have the prescription—the antidote—to self-hatred and to autoimmune disorders. No doctor can give it to you. It is Psalm 139. Read it. Read all of it. Read it over and over and over again until you embrace its truth from your heart. You will find yourself and how God thinks about you in Psalm 139. Below is just a portion of it.

> *For thou hast possessed my reins: thou hast covered me in my mother's womb. I will praise thee; for I am fearfully and wonderfully made: marvellous are thy works; and that my soul knoweth right well. My substance was not hid from thee, when I was made in secret, and curiously wrought in the lowest parts of the earth. Thine eyes did see my substance, yet being unperfect; and in thy book all my members were written, which in continuance were fashioned, when as yet there was none of them. How precious also are thy thoughts unto me, O God! How great is the sum of them! If I should count them, they are more in number than the sand: when I awake, I am still with thee.*   (Psalm 139:13–18)

Embrace the truth of Psalm 139 that you are *"fearfully and wonderfully made"* and that His thoughts toward you are precious and more in number than the sand! Repent for hating and rejecting yourself to this God who loves you. Stop this self-accusation.

The enemy is the accuser of the brethren! Why would you believe the enemy instead of believing the living God and what He says in Psalm 139? Satan poisoned you. I'm giving you the antidote. I'm giving you the Word of God so that you will be delivered and healed.

If you don't agree with God, if you don't believe the truth of His Word, you are in self-idolatry. You see yourself as your own counselor; you see yourself as knowing more than God. You become the source of your own identity. But the Father knew you before you were born, while you were still in your mother's womb. You are no accident.

God sent his Holy Spirit specially to gather you to Himself through Jesus's atonement, and you responded, "Yes." Now you need to embrace that message of salvation and what it means for you each and every day. When you were born again, you became a son or daughter of the Father of all spirits. (See Hebrews 12:9.) Why would you doubt Him now? *"What shall we then say to these things? If God be for us, who can be against us?"* (Romans 8:31).

Let God be true in your life! I don't care what your mother or father said to you. I don't care if you were put up for adoption. I don't care if you were an orphan. You're not an orphan anymore! God has adopted you as His own! *"For ye have not received the spirit of bondage again to fear; but ye have received the Spirit of adoption, whereby we cry, Abba, Father"* (Romans 8:15). Quit arguing that point with God. You do not have to suffer self-accusation any longer! If you will believe God's Word, you will be set free!

WHAT'S NEXT?

Bless the LORD, O my soul, and forget not all his benefits:
who forgiveth all thine iniquities;
who healeth all thy diseases.
—Psalm 103:2–3

We have taken a journey together to expose the spiritual roots of diseases through the knowledge of biblical truth. Let's review a few of these foundational truths concerning the healing of disease.

First, spiritually rooted disease is a result of separation from God, separation from yourself, or separation from others. Therefore, all healing of spiritually rooted diseases begins with reconciliation with God—receiving His love, embracing Him as your Father, and making your peace with Him. Reconciliation with yourself and with others are the next essential steps.

Second, we recognize that there are two kingdoms waging war on the inside of us: the law of sin and the law of God. Remember, the apostle Paul expressed our need to be set free from the temptations and the root of sin in our lives through Jesus Christ: *"O wretched man that I am! who shall deliver me from the body of this death? I thank God through Jesus Christ our Lord"* (Romans 7:24–25).

Third, once we are delivered from these roots, it becomes our responsibility to renew our minds and change those old patterns of ungodly thinking. Casting down evil imaginations and filling yourself with the Word of God in your thought life is your responsibility. *"Casting down imaginations, and every high thing that exalteth itself against the knowledge of God, and bringing into captivity every thought to the obedience of Christ"* (2 Corinthians 10:5).

At Be in Health, we call this process Walk Out. We even have a retreat called Walk Out Workshop, or WOW, because we know how important it is to walk out the process of our sanctification and stay on track with the biblical truths that set us free from disease.

THE 8 RS TO FREEDOM

We also teach what we call the "8 Rs to Freedom."[14] It's vital for you to remember and apply these principles. Post them where you can see them daily, such as on your refrigerator or your

---

14. See Henry W. Wright, *A More Excellent Way* (New Kensington, PA: Whitaker House, 2009), 161–169.

bathroom mirror. Mostly important, post them on your heart. They are the pathway to your freedom!

1. **Recognize.** *You must recognize what it is.* Recognize the root problem(s) in your life: bitterness, hatred, fear, anxiety, anger, hostility, self-hatred, etc. Pray for discernment from the Holy Spirit. Discern good from evil in your life.

2. **Responsibility.** *You must take responsibility for what you recognize.* Not everybody wants to take responsibility after they recognize the problem. You need to take responsibility. God will walk alongside you, but He won't do it for you!

3. **Repent.** *Repent to God for participating in what you recognize.* The Bible tells us, *"Repent ye therefore, and be converted, that your sins may be blotted out, when the times of refreshing shall come from the presence of the Lord"* (Acts 3:19). Some people get mad at me when I tell them they need to repent to be free from disease. If you go to a doctor to find out why you are sick and how to get better, would you be offended if he told you the truth? Then, please, do not be offended if I tell you the truth. I love you, and I care what happens to you. I'm teaching you how to defeat evil spirits and disease.

4. **Renounce.** *You must make what you recognize your enemy and renounce it.* To repent literally means "to turn away from." Consider your past root of sin as your enemy, and renounce it! Some people have remorse, but they do not change on the inside. They

don't turn away from their sin. But I want you to get away from evil—as fast as you can. Love yourself, but hate the evil!

5. **Remove it. *Get rid of it, once and for all!*** Say to the law of sin within you, "Not only do I renounce you, but you and I cannot exist at the same place and the same time together." *"Cast away from you all your transgressions, whereby ye have transgressed; and make you a new heart and a new spirit"* (Ezekiel 18:31). Get that law of sin out of your face, and let God give you a new heart and spirit.

6. **Resist. *When it tries to come back, resist it!*** James 4:7 tells us that we are to submit ourselves to God and resist the devil: *"Submit yourselves therefore to God. Resist the devil, and he will flee from you."* Which one comes first? Submitting to God. Only then will you have the power to resist the enemy, not before. Whatever you have dealt with will try to come back. That is why we need God and each other to resist it.

7. **Rejoice. *Give God thanks for setting you free.*** Give God glory for your freedom! Praise Him that you have experienced grace and mercy from a living God who loves you. He is worthy of your praise!

8. **Restore. *Help someone else get free.*** After you have received the blessings of God, it's time for you to begin helping to restore others. Part of restoring is bringing the gospel to those you love, instructing those who are separated from the refreshing of the Lord, and

discipling them in freedom from disease. *"That there should be no schism in the body; but that the members should have the same care for one another. And whether one member suffer, all the members suffer with it; or one member be honoured, all the members rejoice with it"* (1 Corinthians 12:25–26).

CHANGED INTO GOD'S IMAGE

Never forget that you are being changed into God's image as you follow His Word. *"But we all, with open face beholding as in a glass the glory of the Lord, are changed into the same image from glory to glory, even as by the Spirit of the Lord"* (2 Corinthians 3:18). Don't let anyone steal the truths that you have learned here. People with unbelief will try to debate you, discourage you, and drag you down to their image. You are not being formed into the image of any other person! You're being transformed into the image of God! As you are being changed into His image, you can expect Him to heal you of the diseases of the enemy because God honors His Word and His image. He honors who He is in you, not at the head level but at the heart level.

Through Jesus Christ, the Father is recapturing and recovering what He lost in the tragedy of the garden of Eden—His image in mankind. You are a product of that recovery and restoration. You are being called out of darkness and being changed into His marvelous light. *"But ye are a chosen generation, a royal priesthood, an holy nation, a peculiar people; that ye should shew forth the praises of him who hath called you out of darkness into his marvellous light"* (1 Peter 2:9). But you cannot be transformed unless you are reformed by the Word, because *"faith cometh by an holy hearing, and hearing by the Word of God"* (Romans 10:17).

FOLLOW THROUGH TO DEFEAT THE ENEMY!

I want to encourage you to follow through with your complete freedom from disease. Don't let the enemy discourage you. Everybody wants to be prayed for, but not everyone will follow up by defeating the lies of the enemy and embracing God's truth. Remember this Scripture: *"Ye shall know the truth, and the truth shall make you free"* (John 8:32). What I have been teaching you is designed to give you the truth and the faith to believe. This is not blind faith but real faith based on the knowledge of a living God revealed in the Bible. Your freedom was paid for over two thousand years ago on the cross, and the power of God was released into your life so that you could live in freedom. The Creator of the universe—your heavenly Father—wants you to be free!

> *Before I formed thee in the belly I knew thee; and before thou camest forth out of the womb I sanctified thee.*
>
> (Jeremiah 1:5)

> *But now thus saith the LORD that created thee, O Jacob, and he that formed thee, O Israel, Fear not: for I have redeemed thee, I have called thee by thy name; thou art mine.*
>
> (Isaiah 43:1)

Receive this prayer:

Father, I come to You in the name of Jesus. I want to thank You for those who have taken the time to read this book. I know from Psalm 139 in Your Word that they are fearfully and wonderfully made, and Your hand is upon each and every one of them. I know that I have given them many things to think about from Your Word. I ask You to release Your Holy Spirit to bring understanding and conviction, so that they may be changed from the inside out, and that diseases would vanish.

Father, we are just people, men and women from many different backgrounds. We have listened to lies we didn't know were lies; we have pursued courses we thought were right but are leading to our destruction. Please show us the good way where there is rest for our souls. Teach us to grow up in this thing called life and mature as sons and daughters of God. Let this be, Father, so that we may be whole in spirit, soul, and body, and that the generations after us would also be whole and a light to the world of Your glory and goodness and love toward us. Thank You so much for Your mercy, Sir, and continue to teach us by Your grace. In Jesus's name I pray. Amen.

WHAT BE IN HEALTH OFFERS

Now that we've exposed the spiritual roots of autoimmune diseases, you may be interested in these other resources that Be in Health® has to offer:

FOR MY LIFE®

For My Life is a one-week retreat hosted by Be in Health at our campus in Thomaston, Georgia. It is designed to help people who are seeking healing and restoration of their physical, emotional, and spiritual health. We believe that most diseases result from separation in relationship from God, ourselves, and others. This retreat will help you to identify and deal with the root issues that may be keeping you from being in health.

The For My Life retreat consists of intensive teachings, group ministry sessions, time to interact with the teachers and ask questions, and a time for personal prayer for healing at the end of the week. Be in Health endeavors to make For My Life a safe place for you to find hope and healing for your life.

WALK OUT® WORKSHOP (WOW)

After For My Life, the next step is the Walk Out Workshop (WOW). The term "walk out" refers to the journey of walking out of the old life of disease and hopelessness and entering into a new life of health and wholeness. During this one-week workshop, our team and attendees roll up their sleeves and begin to get really interactive with the principles from For My Life.

We address topics such as how to not go into guilt when we fall short, becoming established in our identity, overcoming temptation, how to forgive when you've been hurt, and learning to walk in the Father's love. Break-out groups, lots of Q & A, and continued healing of your spirit, soul, and body are all part of this amazing week.

FOR MY LIFE® EXPANDED (4MLX)

The For My Life eXpanded Retreat is our brand-new, next in series, five-day retreat, which will take you even deeper into the Be in Health teachings. Develop a profound understanding of the specific spiritual roots of major disease classes and discover powerful insights into healing and recovery in God. This retreat will set you on the next level of your overcomer journey. There are also corporate times of ministry throughout the week.

FOR MY LIFE® KIDS AND FOR MY LIFE® YOUTH

Every year in June and July, we offer For My Life for the whole family; that is the For My Life Adult, For My Life Youth (ages 13–17), and For My Life Kids (ages 6–12) Retreats all in the same week! This is an opportunity for the whole family to be transformed and healed from the inside out.

We hear so many people say, "If only I had known this when I was younger, I would have been saved from so much torment and heartache!" We've listened and developed these specialized retreats to continue our mission of establishing generations of overcomers. In the For My Life family week, everybody in the family can benefit and be on the same page spiritually. We take the same information that is presented in the adult For My Life Retreat but reformat it to be relevant and engaging for each audience.

WOW KIDS

After the For My Life family weeks, we have the WOW family weeks. This is an opportunity for the whole family to come and learn how to be overcomers together. The WOW Kids class (ages 6–12) will equip your children with the skills that they need to be overcomers. With a fun, engaging format, games, activities, and special "tools for freedom," your kids are sure to have a blast, make lasting memories, make new friends, and come out with valuable resources that will help them on their overcomer journey throughout their lives.

 To learn more about the Be in Health Retreats, visit: www.beinhealth.com/for-my-life

THE OVERCOMERS' COMMUNITY®

The journey of being an overcomer can be challenging, and we don't want you to have to do it alone. That is why we've developed the Overcomers' Community. This is a membership-based online forum dedicated to being a safe place for you to connect with the Be in Health Team as well as with other overcomers. You can ask questions, get support and encouragement, share testimonies, find specific spiritual roots of diseases, have access to a wide selection of complete teachings, access our private Facebook page, and more! We look forward to joining you and assisting you in your walk-out journey. With God's help, we can do this together!

 To learn more about the Overcomers' Community, visit: www.beinhealth.com/ overcomers-community

BE IN HEALTH® CONFERENCES NEAR YOU

Our Be in Health Team travels too! We bring one- to three-day conferences to locations all over the world. If you want to find out more about these conferences and when one might be held in your area, or if you are interested in helping us bring a conference to your area, go to: www.beinhealth.com

SPIRITUAL LIFELINE®

Spiritual Lifeline is a ministry of love and personal assistance from the Be in Health team; it is our most individualized form of ministry to you. Our Father promises to deliver us from the enemy as we apply His Word. Together, we'll look at God's plan for your situation and His promises that will sustain you. Private ministry and prayer sessions are provided over the phone or through an online voice- or video-calling platform.

Spiritual Lifeline is not a starting place at Be in Health. It is designed to come alongside and assist those who have previously attended our For My Life Retreat or have read and are applying the principles of Dr. Wright's books *A More Excellent Way* and *Exposing the Spiritual Roots of Disease*.

To learn more about Spiritual Lifeline visit: www. beinhealth.com/phone-ministry

HEALTH RESOURCES

You can find all the information that we offer on specific disease and mental health topics. Under each topic, all the relevant Be in Health teachings, conferences, blogs, YouTube videos, healing testimonies, and related resources are categorized so you can find everything you need in one place. We continue to add new content, so keep checking back for more of the information you are looking for!

Discover our Health Resources at: www.beinhealth. com/healing-resources

BE IN HEALTH® BOOKSTORE

If you enjoyed this book, you will love our other books and teaching resources in the Be in Health Bookstore. You will find an extensive selection of materials by Dr. Henry W. Wright, Pastor Donna Wright, and other leadership team members.

Topics range from the possible spiritual roots of diseases to how to overcome specific spiritual issues to teachings on sound biblical doctrine.

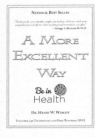

Dr. Henry W. Wright's book *A More Excellent Way* is our number one resource, selling over 300,000 copies worldwide. It is an excellent, comprehensive introduction to the root causes behind diseases and how to overcome them in your life. Included in the back of the book are 150 healing testimonies and a free teaching DVD.

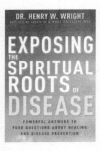

In *Exposing the Spiritual Roots of Disease*, Dr. Wright presents a thoroughly biblical and compelling case for healing. If you think you've read all you need to know about healing, it's time to take another look! Dr. Wright clearly shows that disease is not a random occurrence and that science and medicine have their place in dealing with illness but can only offer disease management. What if the answers to true healing have been in the Bible all along?

Find these books and more in the Be in Health Bookstore: resources.beinhealth.com

BE IN HEALTH® BLOG

The Be in Health Blog offers biblical insights in a selection of articles about spiritual principles, overcoming, roots to diseases, and more. In addition, there are inspiring testimonies that are sure to encourage you in your own overcoming journey.

Find our blog at: www.beinhealth.com/blog

HOPE OF THE GENERATIONS CHURCH

Be in Health is a ministry of Hope of the Generations Church (HOGC), a local body of believers located in Thomaston, Georgia. HOGC is a nondenominational church and follows the model of the first-century church that was set in place by the apostles. We believe that every church, regardless of its background or diversity, should witness the same things recorded in the Bible: signs, wonders, healings, and miracles. These are life-altering tools of God to establish the authenticity of His Word.

Join us Sunday mornings at 10:00 a.m. EST or Friday nights at 7:00 p.m. EST.

We also stream our church services on our YouTube channel: www.youtube.com/beinhealth

A.C.T.S. GLOBAL:
ASSOCIATION OF CHURCHES TEACHING AND SERVING®

Have you considered that God may be calling you to start, pastor, and establish a local church or gathering? Have the teachings of Be in Health opened your eyes, and now you want to tell others? Do you love people and want to see God's best for their lives?

Do you have a desire to guard the purity of the Bible and share that with others? Do you already, or do you desire to, gather people together to grow, heal, and fellowship together?

Do people come to you for help and direction for their lives? Are you ready to be a pastor but are held back by a lack of resources and training?

If you answered yes to one or more of these questions, A.C.T.S. Global is here to help you take the next step.

 To learn more about A.C.T.S. Global visit: www.actsglobal.com

BE IN HEALTH® E-MAIL LIST

Do you want to stay connected with Be in Health and receive updates, messages from our pastors, news, events, and blog posts directly in your inbox?

 Sign up for Be in Health's mailing list at: www.beinhealth.com

SOCIAL MEDIA

You can also follow us on your favorite social media platform!

Facebook: @beinhealth

Instagram: beinhealth

Twitter: @BeinHealth

YouTube: www.youtube.com/beinhealth

Pinterest: bnhealth

ABOUT THE AUTHOR

Dr. Henry W. Wright (1944–2019) was the senior pastor of Hope of the Generations Church in Thomaston, Georgia, and the president and founder of Be in Health® Global. Be in Health is a ministry that teaches on the spiritual roots of disease and blocks to healing, and hosts the world-renowned For My Life® Retreat.

Wright presented conferences worldwide and across broad denominational lines for over twenty-five years. Recognized for his understanding of disease from a spiritual perspective, he was a frequent guest on many well-known television and radio programs.

Wright was exposed to the power of God's healing at an early age when his mother was miraculously cured of terminal cancer and a fatal tumor that was wrapped around her jugular vein. Paralyzed and dying, she was carried to a church service where she cried out to God for healing so that she could raise her son. She repented of bitterness and made a Hannah-type covenant that she would raise him in the knowledge of God if

He would heal her. God healed her instantly and completely, breaking a genetic pattern of cancer that had been present in her family for generations.

Wright was committed to the belief that human problems are fundamentally spiritual, with associated physical and psychological manifestations. With his insights into the medical as well as the spiritual aspects of disease, he brought a fresh perspective to the process of ministering to the sick. He applied these principles successfully in bringing God's healing to people with a broad range of diseases, many of which were considered incurable.

Under the leadership of his wife, Pastor Donna Wright, and the elders of Hope of the Generations Church, Be in Health continues to carry on Dr. Wright's vision and ministry.